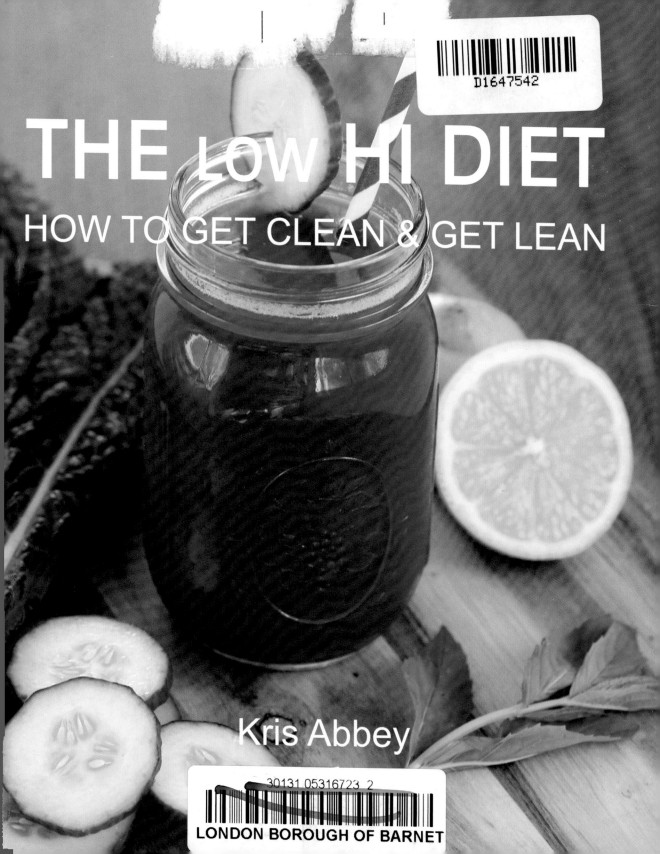

THE LOW HI DIET

HOW TO GET CLEAN & GET LEAN

Kris Abbey

First published in 2014 by New Holland Publishers Pty Ltd
London • Sydney • Auckland

The Chandlery Unit 114 50 Westminster Bridge Road London SE1 7QY United Kingdom
1/66 Gibbes Street Chatswood NSW 2067 Australia
218 Lake Road Northcote Auckland New Zealand

www.newhollandpublishers.com

Copyright © 2014 New Holland Publishers Pty Ltd
Copyright © 2014 in text: Kris Abbey
Copyright © 2014 in images: Dreamstime

Images: Dreamstime unless otherwise specified

A record of this book is held at the British Library and the National Library of Australia.

ISBN 9781742575476

Managing director: Fiona Schultz
Publisher: Diane Ward
Project editor: Jodi De Vantier
Designer: Kris Abbey
Typesetting: Peter Gou
Proofreader: Diane Fowler
Production director: Olga Dementiev
Printer: Toppan Leefung Printing (China)
10 9 8 7 6 5 4 3 2 1

Keep up with New Holland Publishers on Facebook
www.facebook.com/NewHollandPublishers

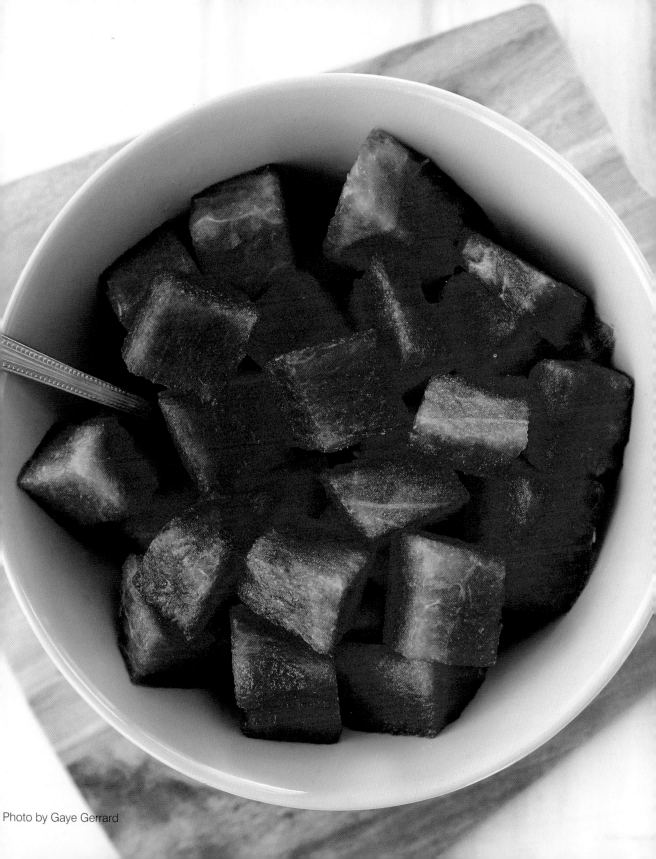

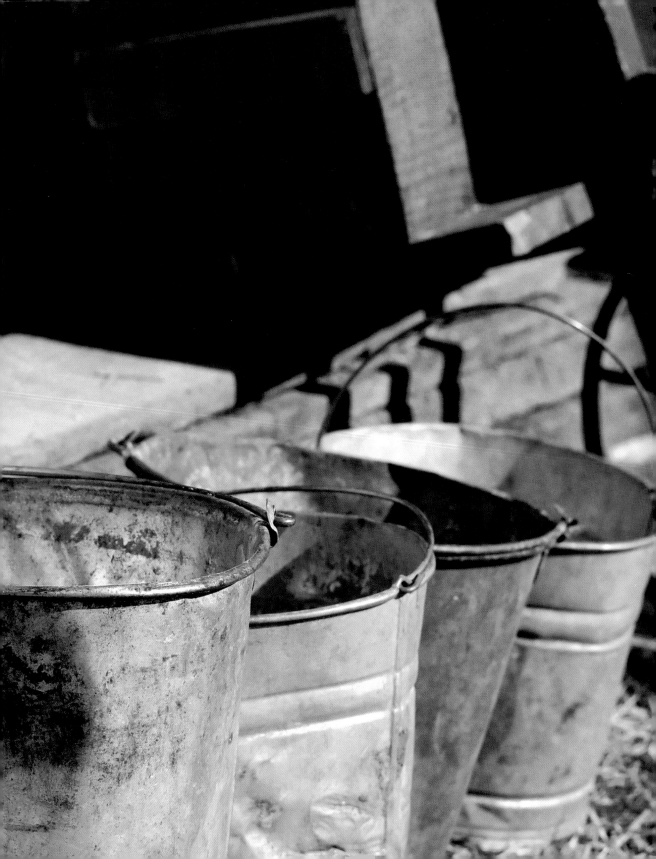

DEDICATION

I dedicate this book to you, for trusting me and allowing me to take these excitng (but sometimes difficult) steps towards better health. Enjoy the journey, and hopefully the destination will be a very healthy, long, long way away.

I also have to pay tribute to my mum and dad (Robyn and Barry Toole), who gave me the most idyllic childhood filled with great memories of good food shared with even better people. My appreciation for the country, all things home-grown and fresh, clean air comes from 'Chicquita' Wirrinya, a little dot on the map but a large place in my heart.

And of course my family, Alan, Isabel, Will and Elise for being the inspiration for so many things!

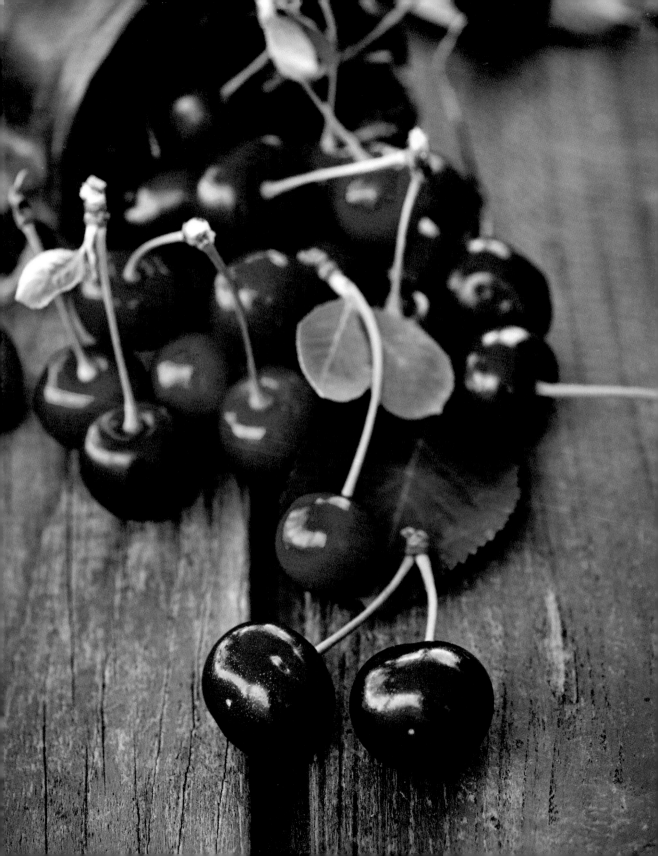

CONTENTS

MY MANIFESTO

EAT WELL

SMILE

Drink two litres of filtered water **EVERY DAY**

SURRENDER

BREATHE

Get plenty **OF SLEEP** each night

DO WORK YOU LOVE

Do something you've been putting off

Take time out just for you

Treasure your **HEALTH**

SURROUND yourself with positive people

Hug more, Give more
COMPLAIN LESS

Understand you can't always control what happens to you, but you can **choose the way you react**

Know you are **FANTASTIC**

LISTEN

Have a good **LAUGH**

Go for a **BUSH WALK**

HAVE A Technology-Free DAY

OBSERVE

Do things that make you HAPPY

Do **NOT** Do Guilt

EAT LOW Hi Foods

Have a green juice on a regular basis

Set a goal for today, next week, next year

BELIEVE IN YOURSELF

ENJOY

Move your body **EVERY DAY**

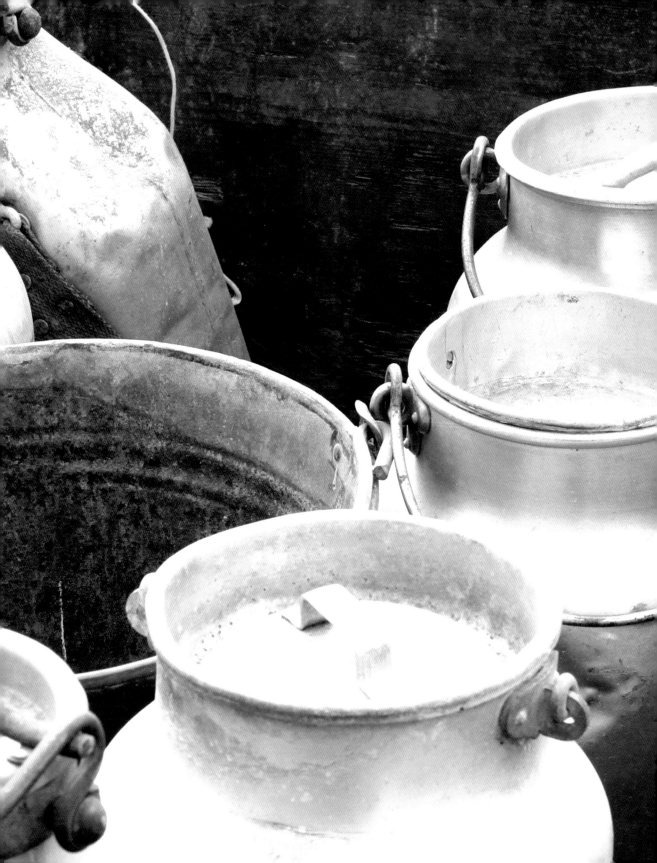

THE BEGINNING

When I started out in the health and wellness industry I was the ripe old age of 15. I used to take the aerobics classes at my school one afternoon a week for the kids who didn't want to do sport. It was compulsory that they do a physical activity so I started out with a smattering of kids in the school gym with ample room for a stretched-out grapevine and a very humble cassette deck playing our music. By the fourth week we had attracted over 90 kids (with a wait list). I was mic'ed up like Madonna to call the instructions with the school AV system supplying the music (which consisted of my mixed tapes recorded from the Top 40 the Sunday night prior). Looking back, my inner devil smiles at the rules we broke—music copyright breaches (allegedly), Occupational Health and Safety and the fact I was just a kid at the school with no formal qualifications (other than a few lessons from my phyiscal education teacher at the time—thank you Jacquie Le Cornu).

Simple times, when rules and red tape didn't ruin a good thing! Just a bunch of kids, who were usually sedentary and possibly lacking confidence, moving and grooving and loving life, and doing something good for their mind, body and soul! The only downside was we didn't have enough room for more kids to participate.

It was circa 1986 when Jane Fonda, Dr Pritikin and Dr Atkins were creeping into our psyche, followed soon by an avalanche of diet books, exercise programs and bright-coloured Lycra workout gear. I couldn't get enough of these people, their books or their videos. Fonda and Pritikin definitely gave me inspiration at that time (Atkins not so much as I had stopped eating red meat!).

But my love of health and wellness didn't actually start at 15. It started a few years prior… I had been a sickly kid … pneumonia, bronchitis, glandular fever and by the time I was 13 I was diagnosed with not one, but two chronic illnesses—Irritable Bowel Syndrome (IBS) and a Hiatus Hernia (which is quite rare in kids, but can happen).

My diet was very healthy—I grew up on a farm and most of what my family ate was home-grown and home-made. My mum is an incredible cook and prepared meals from the ripe vegetables in the garden and meat from our farm. It was literally paddock to plate. I played a lot of sport, so on all accounts I should have been a vital, fit and healthy child.

But something wasn't right. I would get incredible heartburn or severe stomach aches after eating, and the frequency would increase until I was in pain most days. After about three months of doctors and specialists running a large number of non-invasive and invasive tests a diagnosis was made. Back then doctors didn't really know how to treat IBS or hiatus hernias, let alone understand the whys and what for. They simply dealt with the symptoms not the cause.

So I was given a hideous antacid to drink before eating—a sticky liquid chalk that tasted like soap. It was horrendous! Even thinking about it now triggers a gag reflex. I just couldn't do it—it was as bad as the actual symptoms of the illness. It was easier just not to eat. And my already skinny little body became skinnier, and I was becoming less healthy.

My mum (thanks mum) started to seek alternative therapies. Let me paint a picture here. We are talking a good 25 (OK, 30) years ago when naturopaths and yoga teachers were all a bit hoodoo guru and wheat grass was something you gave to cows (and we did). We were country people with little exposure to what was available in this big wide world we live in. The Internet didn't exist in 1983! In my mind (and definitely my mum's) going to see a naturopath slash chiropractor slash acupuncturist was going to be a long shot at best. Although our attitude was we had absolutely nothing to lose and everything to gain.

Well, gain we did. I am happy to say I not only learned what the root cause of my problem was and why I suffered from IBS and a Hiatus Hernia, but also how modifying my diet and lifestyle provided the solution. It allowed me to take control of my condition and lead a pain-free, medicine-free, extremely healthy life! It wasn't a quick fix—in fact it took two visits every week to her practice 62 miles (100 km) away for six months to get 'fixed'. Yet I have stayed symptom-free 25+ years down the track.

At 13 I began learning the principles of food as medicine. I began to understand that many health problems are either caused and/or resolved through our diet and lifestyle. I learnt what foods triggered my underlying hernia and IBS to 'flare up' and I had to eliminate these from my diet. I also had to sleep with a lot of pillows to keep my stomach lower than my oesophagus, but in the scheme of things this certainly beats suffering and taking medication, no question. I will never forget the feeling of being unwell and how feeling well compares. Feeling well and being healthy is definitely the camp I want to be in. For the people out there who are suffering and think it is 'normal', it is not normal! You can (and deserve to) feel energised, vital and healthy; so do not accept anything less.

The foods that gave me the most grief were processed foods such as white bread and pasta, as well as red meat, fried foods and dairy. Since a large part of my diet was meat and dairy (the farm, the cows and all that) it started to make sense as to why I had become so ill and why I had been sick on and off prior to the big crash. My body was constantly trying to deal with something it wasn't able to deal with, and had been doing so for a long time. These foods didn't agree with me but because I kept eating

them, I was putting extra pressure on my immune system, which was always running on empty, or very low at best. So if there was a bug floating around, without a strong immune system to fight it, I'd get sick.

I am using a very basic explanation here and I'm glossing over a cascade of anti-inflammatory and immune responses that occur in your body. However, I am hoping to give you insight into what happens inside your body and each individual cell when it is under stress. Our bodies are an incredible series of complex systems and reactions, all trying to work in harmony so you can go about your business of being and doing, and feeling fabulous while you do so. However, if you put something in the system that compromises this, over time, when your immune system is starting to lose the fight, your body will react.

It could be that certain foods or specific ingredients within a food won't agree with you, so listen when your body is telling you 'that certain food doesn't agree with me!' Your body's voice is generally in the form of pain, bloating, swelling, gas, constipation, diarrhea, headache, runny nose, infection, rashes and the most obvious, weight gain or loss. It can speak many languages! It is a good idea to listen to this voice (or side-effect), as it won't go away until you do something about it. It may even change its tone if you choose to ignore it: like that heartburn might turn up the volume and become a stomach ulcer, and then become something even more sinister. And when I say listen, I mean listen and then act. This is called preventative health!

Learn about what makes you feel sick or unwell. Nine times out of 10 it will be something you eat or drink and the lifestyle you lead. If you want change to happen, you have to change. Stop inflicting the culprit on your body and modify your behaviour.

If you are reading this book I assume it is because you want to get healthy or healthier. I am also guessing you are busy, so I won't mince words or beat around the bush. I apologise if I over-simplify things, however being healthy is simple. You eat nutritious food, you exercise, you feed your passion, and do things that are good for the soul. Unfortunately, over time this simple approach has become confused and complicated. This is due to a lot of reasons—marketing, commercialisation of trends and fads, infiltration of bad food, greed, governments supporting cheap food production, being a time-poor society looking for a quick fix, or being led down the wrong path early in life so bad habits prevail. Now is the time we put the past in the past and get on the path of health and longevity.

You do not want to continue to put a Band Aid over the problem in the hope that it will go away (read: take some medicine to mask the symptoms so you can ignore it for a bit longer). Why not look at your diet and lifestyle and see what you could change that would help improve your health. Maybe it's just cutting back a little of this here or adding a little more of that over there. Today, over 90% of all disease in the Western world is attributable to our lifestyle. Self-inflicted sickness. Come on people, we are better than this.

I believe every cloud does have a silver lining and I truly believe what I went through as a child was a blessing in disguise. It taught me what I need to do to stay healthy and has put me on this incredible journey of preventative health.

From the age of 13, I began learning what food and lifestyle choices my body thrives on and what makes me sick. My hunger for knowledge on the subject was hard to satisfy. I had to read every book on health, and I became obsessed (or blessed) with needing to know all I could on exercise and nutrition. That hunger for knowledge continues to this day.

I love sharing this knowledge and encouraging people like you to restore and treasure your number one asset—your health.

This book is a simple guidebook for health and wellbeing. It isn't anything revolutionary or earth shattering, just a combination of evolution and food from the best natural chef—Mother Earth. I will take you back to basics and put you on the road to great health for good!

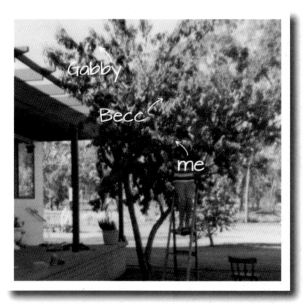

ABOVE: This is me and my two sisters (Gabby & Becc) picking nectarines from the nectarine tree right by our back door. It is the height of summer. I can still taste the super sweet and juicey deliciousness of those nectarines, no refrigerated ripening then!

LET'S GET REAL

This book is a summary of my education, as well as experiences and observations from the last 30 years of working in the health industry. One thing I have learnt, and can assure you of, is the simple fact that diets do not work long-term. If you do a Google search on the word 'diet' you will get about 151 million results. And that doesn't include all the books available on the subject. That's a lot of diets and information (or misinformation) out there. So why are we fatter and sicker than ever? The simple answer ... diets do NOT work!

Sure, you'll lose weight on most diets during the honeymoon period (i.e. the first month or two), but is it a way of eating you can sustain for the rest of your life? Probably not!

Forgive me if you are reading this book under the assumption that it is about a diet. It's not a diet! Eating Low HI is a way of eating healthily that you can enjoy and sustain for the rest of your life. Diet is just that dirty four-letter word I used to lure you in. Sorry, but society has conditioned us to get excited and to think *quick-fix to my weight issues* when we see the word 'diet'. I used it to my advantage. Yes, there is a four-week Get Clean Get Lean program (emphasis on the word program); however, this program is to give your system a clean-up and to reset your default button before embarking on a healthy way of eating for life.

I call this the Low HI Diet. It means eating foods that have had little or no Human Intervention. It is a way of eating that is designed to nourish you for good health and longevity. It's about getting back to basics and eating real food, not the rubbish that has infiltrated our supermarket shelves and is doing damage to your health.

I do 'real' not rules! I will help you to learn about healthy choices and make gradual, lifelong changes that enable you to reach your current and future health goals and then maintain them. For good!

I don't count calories—how tedious! I'd rather you learn to understand good nutrition and listen to your body. Learn to eat when you are hungry and stop when you have had enough. Calories are misleading. Half an avocado and a can of coke may have the same amount of calories, but one is healthy, nourishing and full of natural goodness while the other is not. A calorie doesn't differentiate!

You'll learn to keep portion sizes in control. I've had so many clients tell me they have the healthiest diet on the planet but can't lose weight—then I find out their portion sizes are assuming they are an ultra marathon runner. I want you to learn how much food YOUR body needs (and we are all individual, special people with different needs). For that reason alone, I'm not a fan of the one size fits all approach.

I want to arm you with the tools you need to make the right choices, break bad habits and live a very healthy and fulfilled life. Diets are boring. Life is short. Food is interesting and tasty, and can make you feel so energised if you eat the fresh, full of goodness, low HI variety.

Lastly, diets don't take into account the underlying emotional issues driving us to overeat. By the end of this book I want you to feel so damn good about yourself that you will love yourself and your body to the point you want to cherish and nurture it by feeding it the food it needs to thrive.

I hope you are ready for my revelation that may just stop you from going on a diet ever again. So, let's pull back the curtain and reveal what this book is all about.

I've realised we can cut through the swathe of diets and weight loss *dos and don'ts* and climb this mountain of attaining good health and wellbeing in three easy steps.

STEP 1. GET CLEAN | GET LEAN. I'm not big on the word detox as it can attract a lot of negative attention. Instead let's say cleanse. A regular grease and oil change keeps your car running smoothly. So why not give yourself a grease and oil change, removing the bad and replacing it with the good. I won't lie, it might be tough going, especially if you've been eating a lot of processed food, drinking alcohol and leading a stressful lifestyle. The good news it is over and done with in 28 days. And I can guarantee by the end of it you will feel fantastic!

STEP 2. THE LOW HI WAY OF LIVING. Now that you are all clean and feeling vital we want you to maintain this feeling and eat properly for life. This is where you learn to eliminate or substantially reduce foods that have had a lot of Human Intervention. That is, get rid of food that comes in a box, is full or preservatives or has words in it that don't readily roll off your tongue. Fresh is best, and natural is the new black! Think of the foods your grandparents ate—and I can assure you it wasn't something out of a box. My grandma lived to 99.9 and I would say for the majority of her life, only real food crossed her lips. My nan is a healthy 93 and has a killer veggie patch. She still bakes and cooks all her own meals and I can guarantee you won't find packet food or a commercial sauce in her cupboards—only home-made!

STEP 3. ENJOY LIFE. AGE WELL. Be grateful for all the things your healthy body allows you to do. This is where we take stock and learn that the body isn't just about eating well and exercise. It is also about the stuff we find hard to wrap words around. Happiness, enjoyment, fulfilment and contentment. This is what I call your primary foods—a termed coined by a true pioneer, Joshua Rosenthal! The food that feeds your soul and makes you sing on the inside. It's feeding this primary food that will get you off that diet merry-go-round and stop you from using food to satisfy that something in you that isn't being fed.

That's all there is to it. If you are still reading this, I'd say you're more than ready to take the first step! I'm excited for you, and I know this will be the last 'diet' you will ever do. Let's get going and get you looking and feeling great!

Diet *n.* **1**. a restrictive and boring eating plan; **2**. leaves one feeling hungry and low in energy; **3**. a very vicious cycle; **4**. to be avoided unless it can be sustained for life and fuels your body; **5**. can take the fun out of food.

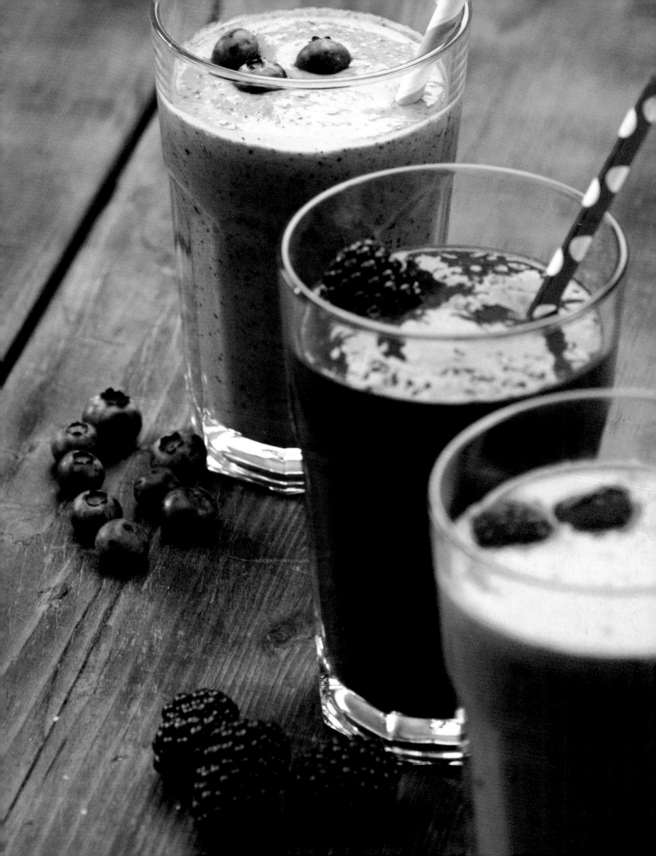

STEP 1
Get Clean | Get Lean

'In order to change we must be sick and tired of being sick and tired.'
Author unknown

DO I NEED A CLEAN?

Your body has its own detoxification system but, like anything, if it is overloaded it begins to fall behind, and the result is a backlog of toxins in the body. The toxins that can't be filtered out of your blood can wreak havoc on your health. And if you're already suffering from an illness, excess toxins can make it worse.

Some of the symptoms of too many toxins in your body are outlined in the box on this page. If you suffer from any of these then you might benefit from a cleanse.

If you experience any of these symptoms, it's your body's way of telling you (very loudly) you need a spring clean. Listen to your body please!

'Today, with more toxins in the environment than ever, it's critical to detox,' says Linda Page, N.D., Ph.D., the author of *Detoxification* (Healthy Healing Publications). Page recommends detoxing for symptoms such as unexplained fatigue, sluggish elimination, irritated skin, allergies or low-grade infections; bags under the eyes; a distended stomach even if the rest of your body is thin; menstrual difficulties; or mental confusion.

Put simply, detoxing (or cleansing) involves giving your body a break from anything toxic, so it can work these excess toxins out of its system. This then gives your immune system a recharge and is ready to fight a good fight again.

Before starting any new eating program it is wise to consult with your health care practitioner. If at any time on the program you experience discomfort, discuss this with your doctor or health care practitioner. It is likely you will get headaches on the first few days, especially if you have a sugar or caffeine addiction. Around day three you might feel a bit down and not really up to being social. These are common withdrawal symptoms. Tissue salts can help alleviate the headaches. As for the low mood, try to ride it out—DO NOT resort to a sugar hit or a glass of wine. Be strong and focus on how fantastic you will feel in a few days. You cannot give up this early in the program.

If you are pregnant, breastfeeding or going through a stressful time, now is not the time to do the program. The program is not recommended for children under the age of 12 or people over 75, or if you suffer from heart disease, or if you are significantly underweight. If you are taking prescribed medication, check with your doctor before starting the program.

Be honest, tick the boxes of anything here you suffer from on a regular basis. You don't have to suffer, you might just need to give you system a good grease and oil change!

- [ ] Frequent headaches
- [ ] Poor digestion and bloating
- [ ] Acne and skin problems
- [ ] Bad breath
- [ ] Feeling sluggish and lacking in energy
- [ ] Poor sleep patterns
- [ ] Muscle aches and pains
- [ ] Inability to concentrate/sense of fogginess
- [ ] Anxiety and/or mood swings
- [ ] Recurring infections
- [ ] Nerve pain or numbess

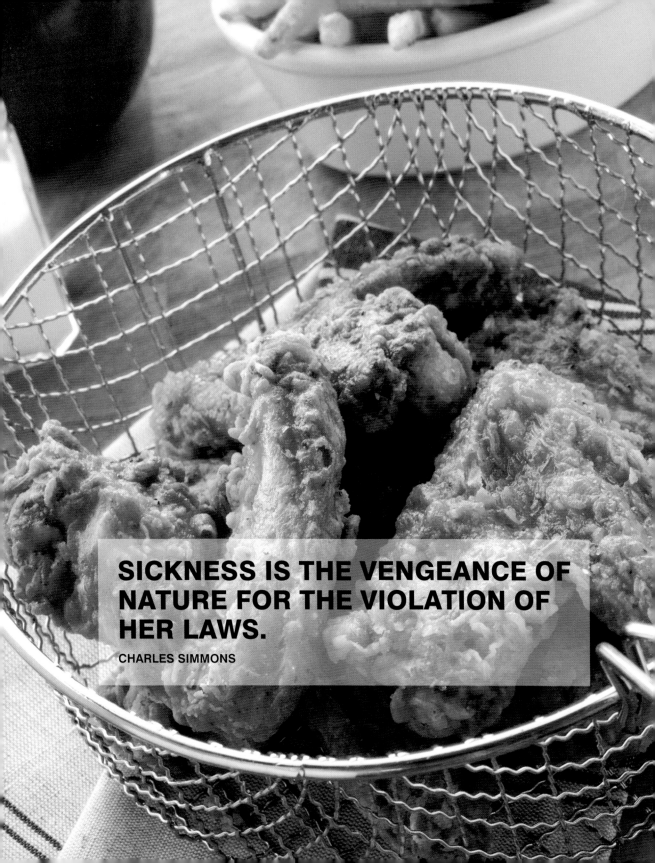

SICKNESS IS THE VENGEANCE OF NATURE FOR THE VIOLATION OF HER LAWS.

CHARLES SIMMONS

YOU ARE WHAT YOU EAT!

Sometimes we live in a state of denial. You might think you are eating healthy, but when you actually take a good hard look at what goes in your mouth, you could be in for a rude shock. There's the sugar in your coffee (and how many of those do you have a day) or that breakfast out of a box that can sit on your pantry shelf for weeks and weeks (nothing vital or fresh there). Not to mention the daily wine with dinner (come on, it's just one, sometimes two) and then the piece of chocolate as you watch TV at night. These are all common habits. They may

have started as an occasional treat but are now habitual behaviours you need to stop, or at least modify so they are occasional again.

I want you to write down absolutely everything you put in your mouth (yep, even the cough drop), as well as drinks (water, soft drinks, juice, hot drinks etc.). Be as honest as you can. It is for your eyes only, and it should highlight the weak points of your day. Knowing when the enemy (cravings) might attack is the best way to be ready to fight it. Plus, doing this exercise often highlights how many toxins we willing put in our body. Time to clean!

	Monday	Tuesday	Wednesday	Thursday	Friday	Saturday	Sunday
Breakfast							
Mid-am							
Lunch							
Mid-pm							
Dinner							
Other							
Drinks							

✳ This form is available for download at krisabbey.com

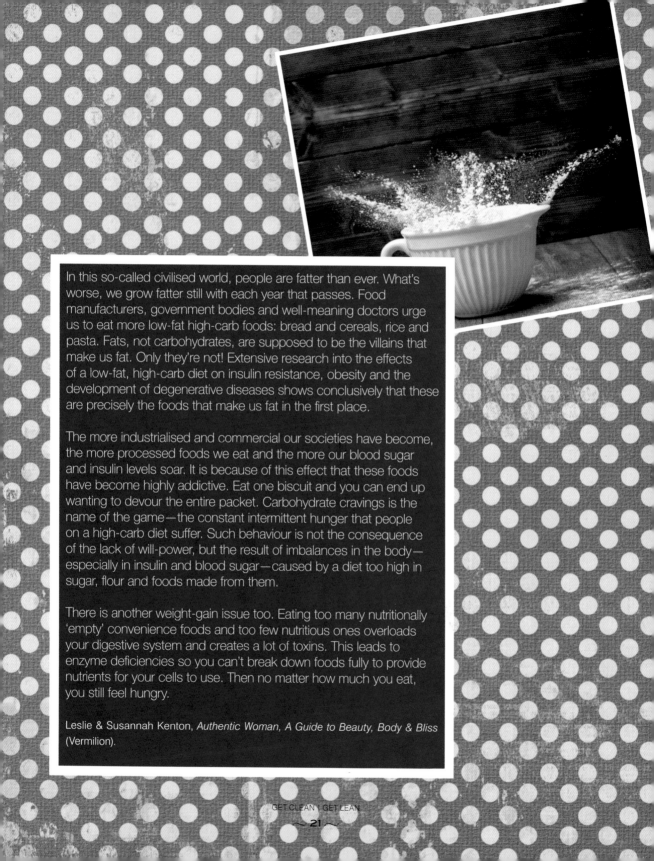

In this so-called civilised world, people are fatter than ever. What's worse, we grow fatter still with each year that passes. Food manufacturers, government bodies and well-meaning doctors urge us to eat more low-fat high-carb foods: bread and cereals, rice and pasta. Fats, not carbohydrates, are supposed to be the villains that make us fat. Only they're not! Extensive research into the effects of a low-fat, high-carb diet on insulin resistance, obesity and the development of degenerative diseases shows conclusively that these are precisely the foods that make us fat in the first place.

The more industrialised and commercial our societies have become, the more processed foods we eat and the more our blood sugar and insulin levels soar. It is because of this effect that these foods have become highly addictive. Eat one biscuit and you can end up wanting to devour the entire packet. Carbohydrate cravings is the name of the game—the constant intermittent hunger that people on a high-carb diet suffer. Such behaviour is not the consequence of the lack of will-power, but the result of imbalances in the body—especially in insulin and blood sugar—caused by a diet too high in sugar, flour and foods made from them.

There is another weight-gain issue too. Eating too many nutritionally 'empty' convenience foods and too few nutritious ones overloads your digestive system and creates a lot of toxins. This leads to enzyme deficiencies so you can't break down foods fully to provide nutrients for your cells to use. Then no matter how much you eat, you still feel hungry.

Leslie & Susannah Kenton, *Authentic Woman, A Guide to Beauty, Body & Bliss* (Vermilion).

WHAT CAN I ACHIEVE?

Reducing your consumption of toxins doesn't have to be a painful or 'scary' task. We have so much fresh food available to us, why would you eat something that has been processed in a lab?

I am a big advocate of Seasonal, Local, Organic and Whole food, prepared with love, and eaten slowly. Food that comes in a packet and can last in the cupboard for months is really stretching the definition of food! I say eat Low HI—food with very little Human Intervention. We will talk more about Low HI later in Step Two.

Simply cutting out processed foods and eating fresh produce will have a marked improvement on your health.

Following the guidelines of the Get Clean Get Lean program (as close as you can) will give your liver, kidneys and lungs a big boost. This will enable them to function better, keeping your blood clean and your body healthy. Think of detoxing like servicing your car. How much smoother does your car run after a service?

At the end of the 4-week Get Clean Get Lean program it is likely you will experience:
* more energy
* more vitality
* loss of fat, not lean muscle tissue
* greater concentration and clarity
* improved skin condition and clearer eyes
* improved digestion
* improved acid/alkaline balance of the body
* improved bowel function
* greater health and wellbeing.

COMMON TOXIC SUBSTANCES:

Truth time. Tick the toxin you are guilty of indulging in on a regular basis. The more ticks, the more you need to do this 28-Day Cleanse.

☐ Alcohol

☐ Sugar

☐ Processed foods

☐ Soft drinks

☐ Caffeine

☐ Artificial colourings, flavourings and sweeteners

☐ Hydrogenated and trans fats

☐ Cigarettes

☐ Drugs

☐ Chemical-based skincare and body products

While you're on the program, try to avoid as many of these toxic substances as you can, if not all of them!

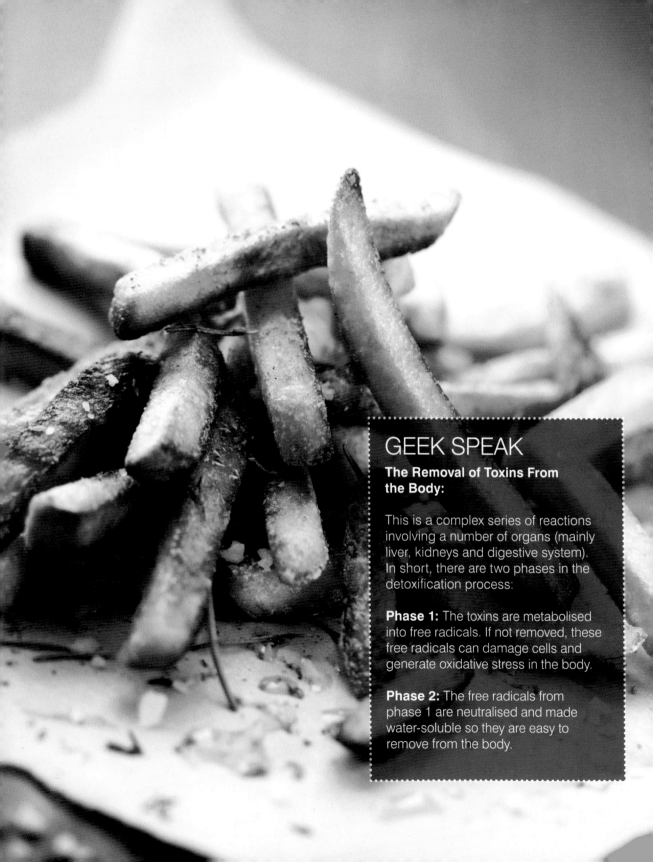

GEEK SPEAK

The Removal of Toxins From the Body:

This is a complex series of reactions involving a number of organs (mainly liver, kidneys and digestive system). In short, there are two phases in the detoxification process:

Phase 1: The toxins are metabolised into free radicals. If not removed, these free radicals can damage cells and generate oxidative stress in the body.

Phase 2: The free radicals from phase 1 are neutralised and made water-soluble so they are easy to remove from the body.

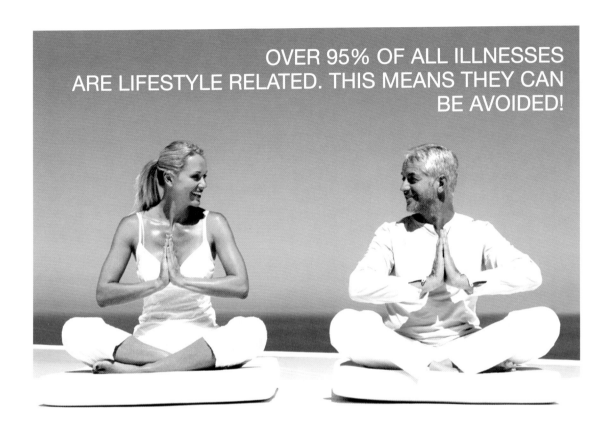

OVER 95% OF ALL ILLNESSES ARE LIFESTYLE RELATED. THIS MEANS THEY CAN BE AVOIDED!

Why am I doing this?

How do I expect to feel at the end?

What is my reward?

GETTING PSYCHED

The word 'detox' has taken such a battering by the media over the past few years that there are more negative connotations and myths associated with it than there are positive ones, such as the wonderful vitality and rejuvenation it can bring to your health. A good detox program can literally be the start of a new lease on life and the essential first step down the path of long-term wellbeing.

Put simply, to detox means to give your blood a good clean (that grease and oil change), which has a profound and positive effect on your liver, kidneys, and every other organ of your body. Our blood accumulates toxins (more than it can filter out) from both external and endogenous (internal) sources. External toxins come into your body through poor diet, drinking too much alcohol, coffee and tea, stress, poor sleep, exposure to environmental toxins (pollution) and taking drugs, among other things. Endogenous sources are usually a result of hormonal or chemical imbalances and by-products of the bacteria in our digestive system. Often excess endogenous toxins are a result of exposure to too many external toxins.

When your blood contains too many toxins it compromises every cell in the body. As a result your health pays a price, and ultimately your hip-pocket does too.

I remember the very first detox program I did, and that intense feeling of being 100 per cent healthy at the end of it. I had spent a week at The Farm at San Benito, Batangas in the Philippines (www.thefarm.com.ph). At the end of the program I had crystal-clear eyes, my skin was glowing and my energy levels were at an all-time high. My usual Irritable Bowel Syndrome symptoms were no more, and I had never felt so vibrant and healthy in my entire life. I remember thinking everyone should experience this feeling. Nirvana!

And yes, I confess that a medically supervised detox program in a beautiful spa environment, with food and juices prepared for you is a great way to detox. However, I also believe that with enough motivation, commitment and advance preparation you can complete a very effective detox program in the comfort of your own home.

So, taking the best bits from some of the wonderful spas around the globe (who have also shared some of their most popular recipes), expert advice from a number of highly regarded naturopaths and nutritionists, combined with my first-hand experience, I have created the Get Clean Get Lean program.

Before you embark, think about why you are doing this program. Is it to re-energise? Lose weight? Undo some of the damage done over the holidays? Or to kick-start a new, healthy lifestyle? Whatever your reasons, write it down. When temptation rears its ugly head, come back to *why* you are doing this. I'm sure the reason *why* is much more meaningful to you than any temptation put before you.

Also think about your end goal. Write that down too. How will it feel to achieve that goal? And what is your reward? Come on, we all need a deal sweetener! A little motivation to keep us on track. What will you reward yourself with (other than health and vitality) at the end of this program? Make it good—you deserve it!

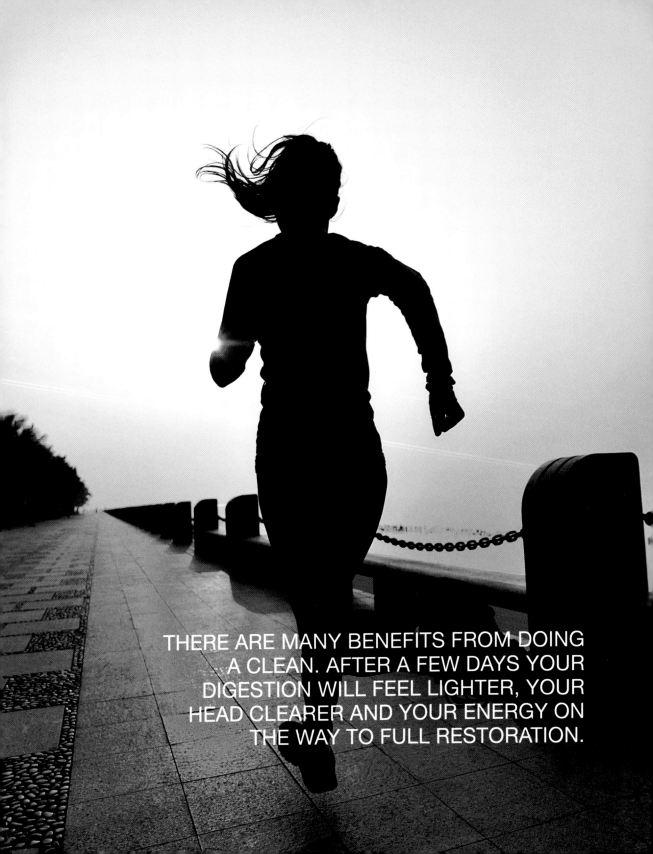

THERE ARE MANY BENEFITS FROM DOING A CLEAN. AFTER A FEW DAYS YOUR DIGESTION WILL FEEL LIGHTER, YOUR HEAD CLEARER AND YOUR ENERGY ON THE WAY TO FULL RESTORATION.

CLEAN AND LEAN

Although this is not a fat loss diet, rather a cleanse, one of the beautiful side-effects is that you will lose fat. Yes fat! You don't want to lose lean muscle tissue or too much fluid. One of the biggest criticisms of fad 'detox' diets is that they encourage the loss of lean muscle tissue, not fat. So, even though you may lose weight on one of those fad detox diets, the weight you are losing is unlikely to be fat, more likely to be lean muscle tissue and water!

Provided you eat protein at every meal, don't starve yourself, and enjoy some exercise (preferably with some form of resistance), you will lose fat, not lean muscle tissue, on the four-week Get Clean Get Lean program. The more lean muscle you have, the faster your metabolism, so it is important to preserve your lean muscle mass.

Toxins love fat. When toxins aren't removed from your body they are stored in the liver or adipose (fat) tissue. Without going into too much detail, while you have an excess of toxins in your body you will have fat! Ironically, a lot of diets suggest special 'diet' food. There's really nothing special about diet food that comes in a box with copious amounts of chemicals added to give it flavour, or synthetic nutrients to replace those denatured during the manufacturing process. They are still processed foods that generate toxins in your body. Fresh is best. Simple!

The aim of detoxifying is to increase the function of your eliminatory organs (liver, kidneys, colon and skin) as well as drawing stored toxins out of cells. Even though exercise is an important part of wellbeing, during this program adequate rest is just as necessary to stimulate and complete the cleansing process. If you over-exercise or place other stresses on your body without getting adequate rest and recovery, the release of toxins will overtake their elimination, which leads to recirculation into the bloodstream. This inevitably leads to headaches, tiredness, skin breakouts or rashes, nausea, cramping and decreased immunity to the point where a cold or flu can take hold.

Detoxification is about resting, cleaning and nourishing the body from the inside out. By removing and eliminating toxins, then feeding your body with healthy nutrients, a good cleanse can help protect you from disease and renew your ability to maintain optimum health. Understanding proper nutrition can be tough when you're given so much misinformation. The next few chapters are dedicated to holistic, real, fundamental nutrition. Understanding this will set you up not only a good cleanse, but a healthy life—for life!

THERE'S REALLY NOTHING SPECIAL ABOUT DIET FOOD THAT COMES IN A BOX WITH COPIOUS AMOUNTS OF CHEMICALS ADDED TO GIVE IT FLAVOUR, OR SYNTHETIC NUTRIENTS TO REPLACE THOSE DENATURED DURING THE MANUFACTURING PROCESS. THEY ARE STILL PROCESSED FOODS THAT GENERATE TOXINS IN YOUR BODY. BETTER IN THE BIN THAN YOUR BODY!

NUTRITION IN A NUTSHELL

For some reason eating a well-balanced diet seems to elude us. If we were all able to complete this simple task, the health of the Western world would be much greater than it is, and the national health bill much lower. All these lifestyle-related diseases such as obesity, cardiovascular disease, type 2 diabetes, metabolic disorders and some allergies and cancers could be avoided if we just ate a balanced, less toxic diet and made better lifestyle choices. So, what is a balanced diet?

It is eating a combination of lean, unprocessed protein, low GI carbohydrates, a colourful array of fresh vegetables, and un-saturated fats. I will cover each of these nutrients in more detail shortly.

The easiest and most visual way to ensure you are eating a balanced diet is to keep the food on your plate in the following proportions:

❉ A quarter of each main meal should be lean protein.

❉ A quarter of each meal should be carbohydrate: starchy vegetables or low GI carbohydrates.

❉ Half of each meal should be non-starchy vegetables (colourful greens, carrot, beetroot etc.).

❉ Add a sprinkle of healthy fats (think nuts, seeds, avocado, olive oil, coconut oil etc.).

LEAN PROTEIN

Poultry (no skin) lean red meat, seafood, eggs, dairy products seeds and nuts beans and lentils soy products, some grains

STARCHY VEGETABLES OR LOW GI CARBS

Pumpkin/squash, cooked carrot, swede, parsnip, cooked beetroot, potato, sweet potato, corn and broad beans Low GI carbs: Quinoa, cornmeal, pearl barley, bulgar, brown rice (ideally basmati), couscous, wholemeal pasta

NON-STARCHY VEGETABLES

Alfalfa, asparagus, aubergine, beansprouts, raw beetroot, broccoli, Brussels sprouts, cabbage, raw carrot, cauliflower, celery, courgette, cucumber, endive, fennel, garlic, kale, lettuce, mangetout peas, mushrooms, onions, peas, peppers, radish, rocket, runner beans, spinach, spring onions, tenderstem broccoli, tomatoes, watercress

❉ A similar principle applies to snacks, which should comprise of both protein (for example, 1¾ oz/50 g of nuts or seeds) and low GI carbohydrate (such as berries).

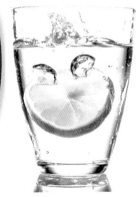

❉ And don't forget your two litres of filtered water each day so you are well hydrated.

PORTION CONTROL TIPS

Have a salad before eating your meal. It will curb your appetite and give you a sense of satiety sooner.

If eating out, split a smaller meal with a friend. Or order two smaller meals, instead of an appetiser and a main. And don't be afraid to ask for small servings. It will save a lot of over-eating or guilt when you leave food on your plate.

Buy or make single serving snacks. You can easily portion out a large container of nuts into smaller individual serving bags. You will be much less likely to go back for an extra bag than an extra handful.

Keep seconds out of sight. Leave the food in the kitchen, and bring your plate to the table. You will usually think twice about getting up from the table to refill your plate, whereas you might be more tempted to dig in again if the food is within arm's reach.

Have healthy snacks between meals. This will keep you satisfied and stop you from overeating at meal times.

PROTEIN

Proteins are the building blocks for life. Brain cells, muscle, skin, hair and nails are just some of the body parts that are protein-based. Protein is an essential part of our diet and foods that contain protein include flesh foods (poultry, beef, lamb and fish), eggs, dairy, nuts, seeds, legumes (beans and lentils) and some grains.

Protein, when digested, is broken down into amino acids, which are chemically linked to each other by peptide bonds. There are about 20 different amino acids that can be put together in different combinations to make up the millions of proteins found in nature. The two broad classes of amino acids are those that can be made by the body (non-essential amino acids) and those that must be supplied through your diet (essential amino acids). The table below outlines some of the food sources providing both types of amino acids.

The amount of protein you need depends on your weight, age and lifestyle. As a rough guide, the recommended dietary intake (RDI) for protein (measured in grams per kilogram/ounces per pound of bodyweight) is:

* 0.75 g per kg (0.012 oz per lb) for adult women
* 0.84 g per kg (0.0135 oz per lb) for adult men
* 1 g per kg (0.016 oz per lb) for pregnant and breastfeeding women, and for men and women over 70.

For example, a 75 kg adult male would need 63 g of protein per day. It is recommended that up to 25 per cent of total energy intake per day is from protein sources. Your body can't store protein and will excrete any excess. Therefore, the most effective way of using the daily protein requirement is to eat small amounts at every meal. Using the example of the 75 kg male above, this would require that he eats approximately 21 g of protein at three meals each day. Most people eat more protein than they need, so deficiencies are rare.

Essential Amino Acids (Complete Proteins)	Non-essential Amino Acids (Incomplete Proteins)
Animal sources such as chicken, beef, lamb, seafood, pork, veal, and turkey Eggs Dairy Plants containing essential amino acids include: soy, quinoa, amaranth seed Since our body cannot make these amino acids (there are nine) it is essential they are supplied through your diet.	Grains Nuts Beans Seeds Peas Corn If you are following a strict vegetarian or vegan diet, combine foods from two or more incomplete proteins to create complete proteins.

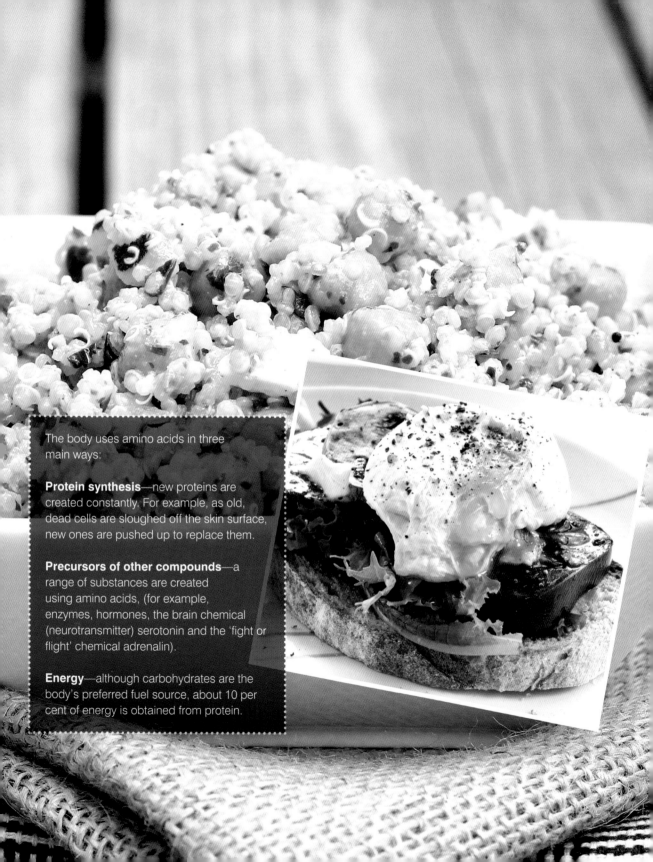

The body uses amino acids in three main ways:

Protein synthesis—new proteins are created constantly. For example, as old, dead cells are sloughed off the skin surface, new ones are pushed up to replace them.

Precursors of other compounds—a range of substances are created using amino acids, (for example, enzymes, hormones, the brain chemical (neurotransmitter) serotonin and the 'fight or flight' chemical adrenalin).

Energy—although carbohydrates are the body's preferred fuel source, about 10 per cent of energy is obtained from protein.

At around 50 years of age you will begin to gradually lose skeletal muscle. This loss is known as sarcopenia, and is common in the elderly. It is also worsened by chronic illness, poor diet or inactivity. Increasing the amount of protein you eat to the upper end of the RDI range, as well as weight bearing exercise, can help maintain muscle mass and strength. This is vital for your ability to stay mobile and reduces your risk of injury.

STRENUOUS EXERCISE & EXTRA PROTEIN

Contrary to popular belief, people who exercise vigorously or are trying to put on muscle mass don't need to consume extra protein. Studies show that weight-trainers who do not eat extra protein (either in food or protein powders) still gain muscle at the same rate as weight-trainers who do supplement their diets with protein. A very high-protein diet can strain the kidneys and liver, and prompt excessive loss of the mineral calcium. The best thing you can do to help improve or maintain muscle mass is to consume protein from your RDI within 30 minutes of exercising. Make this protein source high-quality, lean and combined with a low GI carbohydrate to help maintain your body's protein balance. Studies have shown this to be beneficial, even if exercise is low to moderate intensity aerobic exercise (such as walking). If you can't get the required protein/carb combo into your body through food within 30 minutes, I can recommend the wonderful Clean Lean Protein powder. It is organic, delicious and made from pea protein, so totally fine for vegans and vegetarians. And it's not full of all the manufactured additives of many commercial protein powders. Clean Lean Protein is available through my shop krisabbey.com/shop.

A general guide to healthy eating recommends particular serves per day from the lean meat, poultry, fish, eggs, legumes and beans, and nuts and seeds food category, including:

3 serves for adult men

2½ serves for adult women

2½ to 3½ serves for breastfeeding and pregnant women, and people over 70

A standard serving size is one of:

* 65 g cooked lean red meats
* 80 g cooked poultry
* 100 g cooked fish fillet
* 2 large eggs
* 1 cup cooked dried beans, lentils, chickpeas, split peas or canned beans
* 170 g tofu
* 30 g nuts or seeds
* 250 mL (1 cup) milk
* 200 g (¾ cup) yoghurt
* 40 g (2 slices) hard cheese.

THE PROBLEM PROTEIN

I know of lot of people who suffer from gluten intolerances and coeliac disease. Gluten is a protein found in certain carbohydrates (we will get to carbs shortly). These include wheat, rye, barley, triticale and oats. There is a lot of speculation about the high incidence of gluten intolerances and allergies, and for the most part the food industry have their head in the sand about it. Evidence suggests food processing and manufacturing has evolved quicker than the human body can keep up. It was less than 100 years ago that we started processing wheat for food, prior to that it was rarely eaten, or if it was it was in the form of spelt and emmer—not a bleached white, processed powdery flour. Highly processed grains in general (including wheat) are a relatively new addition to our diet.

For some people, eating or drinking anything containing gluten can cause different types of undesirable reactions. The most extreme of these is the auto-immune condition known as coeliac disease. Some other types of reactions are known as non-coeliac gluten sensitivity, gluten sensitivity, or gluten intolerance. It is important to note that gluten sensitivity is different from a wheat allergy.

People with coeliac disease and gluten sensitivity show improvement when they follow a gluten-free diet. Unfortunately, wheat and gluten have permeated so many products available today you will have to give up a lot more than bread and commercial breakfast cereals. You really have to read labels to ensure gluten is not creeping into your diet through salad dressings, soups, sauces and even chewing gum. Avoid pasta, muffins, pastries, baked goods, couscous, curry powders and seasonings, tomato sauce, margarine, processed and tinned meats, tinned vegetables, MSG and all alcohol made from grains (beer, whiskey, bourbon and liqueurs).

Your diet is better off without these foods anyway, as gluten isn't the only offending ingredient. But all gluten food is off-limits while you are cleansing.

SYMPTOMS OF GLUTEN INTOLERANCE

If you suffer from any of the following symptoms you may have a gluten allergy.

- [ ] Sniffling or sinus problems
- [ ] Fatigue or chronic fatigue syndrome
- [ ] Depression
- [ ] Poor concentration or brain fog
- [ ] Anaemia
- [ ] Diarrhoea or constipation
- [ ] Abdominal bloating
- [ ] Mouth ulcers
- [ ] Crohn's Disease
- [ ] Diverticulitis

Go 10 days without any wheat, barley, rye or spelt and see if symptoms disappear. If they do there is a very strong chance you are gluten intolerant. You can also do a IgG blood test, which can detect the presence of immunoglobulin G, an antibody that would indicate your body sees gluten as an allergen.

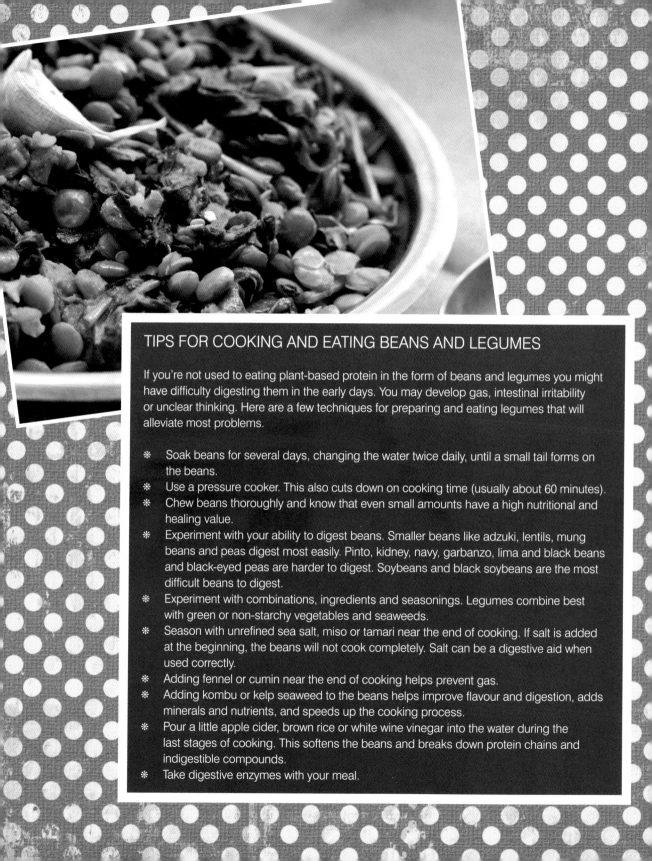

TIPS FOR COOKING AND EATING BEANS AND LEGUMES

If you're not used to eating plant-based protein in the form of beans and legumes you might have difficulty digesting them in the early days. You may develop gas, intestinal irritability or unclear thinking. Here are a few techniques for preparing and eating legumes that will alleviate most problems.

* Soak beans for several days, changing the water twice daily, until a small tail forms on the beans.
* Use a pressure cooker. This also cuts down on cooking time (usually about 60 minutes).
* Chew beans thoroughly and know that even small amounts have a high nutritional and healing value.
* Experiment with your ability to digest beans. Smaller beans like adzuki, lentils, mung beans and peas digest most easily. Pinto, kidney, navy, garbanzo, lima and black beans and black-eyed peas are harder to digest. Soybeans and black soybeans are the most difficult beans to digest.
* Experiment with combinations, ingredients and seasonings. Legumes combine best with green or non-starchy vegetables and seaweeds.
* Season with unrefined sea salt, miso or tamari near the end of cooking. If salt is added at the beginning, the beans will not cook completely. Salt can be a digestive aid when used correctly.
* Adding fennel or cumin near the end of cooking helps prevent gas.
* Adding kombu or kelp seaweed to the beans helps improve flavour and digestion, adds minerals and nutrients, and speeds up the cooking process.
* Pour a little apple cider, brown rice or white wine vinegar into the water during the last stages of cooking. This softens the beans and breaks down protein chains and indigestible compounds.
* Take digestive enzymes with your meal.

KEEPING IT CLEAN

Just to recap, you need protein for repair and maintenance of your cells, for certain reactions in your body and occassionally for energy. You should eat about 75 g (but no more than 100 g) per day.

While you are on the Get Clean Get Lean program, the main source of protein will come from plants, nuts, seeds and grains, like quinoa (pronounced keen-wah). Animal sources of protein are harder to digest and produce more toxins than plant-based proteins, which is why you will limit them while you're trying to reduce your toxic load and clean your system. If you must eat meat, make it lean and organic if possible, and keep the portion size to no larger than your fist. A little bit later on in this section, I outline protein and portion size recommended while you are on the program, but here is a little taste to whet your appetite:

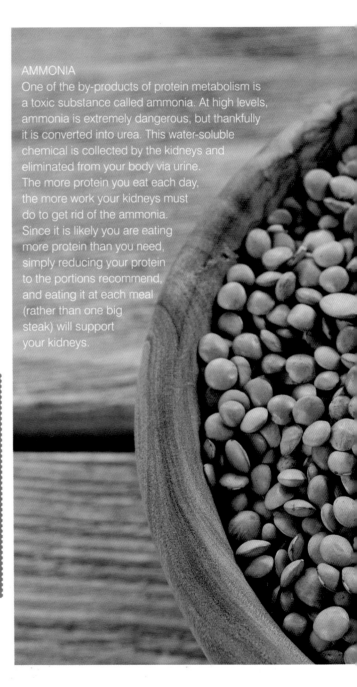

AMMONIA

One of the by-products of protein metabolism is a toxic substance called ammonia. At high levels, ammonia is extremely dangerous, but thankfully it is converted into urea. This water-soluble chemical is collected by the kidneys and eliminated from your body via urine. The more protein you eat each day, the more work your kidneys must do to get rid of the ammonia. Since it is likely you are eating more protein than you need, simply reducing your protein to the portions recommend, and eating it at each meal (rather than one big steak) will support your kidneys.

PERFECT PROTEIN PORTIONS

- Eat three servings of either quinoa, beans, tofu (organic), lentils, nuts or seeds every day.

- Occasionally replace one of these servings with animal protein (meat, fish, poultry or eggs); however, ensure it is lean, free-range and/or organic.

- Limit meat to three times per week.

CARBOHYDRATES

Carbohydrate is the primary source of energy for your body and its functions, since it is simpler to metabolise than fats or amino acids. All carbohydrates are broken down into glucose by the body. The more simple the carbohydrate, the quicker it is converted to glucose, causing an influx of glucose in the blood. This creates a spike in the levels of blood sugar (or blood glucose).

Your body reacts to bring blood sugar levels back to a normal level by producing insulin (a hormone secreted by the pancreas). Insulin helps convert the blood sugar to glycogen, where it is stored in the muscles and tissues. Once these stores are full, the excess blood sugar is converted to fat. Read that sentence again. Yes, converted to fat. But hang on, it's a carbohydrate not a fat!

And that has been where society has gone wrong since the 1980s with the introduction of 'diet' food and low-fat diets. Diets aimed to cut calories—usually by cutting fat, since fat has the most calories per gram. On paper that would be the logical thing to do; however, without fully understanding the complexities of fat and carbohydrate metabolism the reality hasn't been as good as the theory. Again, I'll remind you that all calories are not equal; there's a bit more to it than that. By reducing fat and replacing it with refined, high GI carbohydrates to give it flavour, diet food manufacturers have in fact made you fatter. Good for business I guess!

Complex carbohydrates have a less dramatic effect on blood sugar levels, and consequently on insulin, because they take much longer to be metabolised and are consequently, released more slowly into our blood. They also keep you satisfied for longer.

Carbohydrates are now classified according to their Glycaemic Index (GI) or the effect they have on blood sugar. Simple carbohydrates have a high

LOW GI CARBOHYDRATES

Breads—multigrain, soy and linseed, heavy fruit breads, sourdough
Grains—brown and wild rice, quinoa, other whole grains, tabouli, pearl barley, wholewheat pasta, oats, unsweetened muesli, high-fibre wheat bran cereal
Vegetables—sweet potato, okra, mushrooms, peas, beans, broccoli, artichoke, eggplant
Fruit—apples, oranges, pears, mandarins, grapefruit, bananas
Other—raw honey, soya products

HIGH GI CARBOHYDRATES

Breads—white bread
Grains—short grain rice, toasted rice cereal, pasta
Vegetables—instant potato, tomatoes, lettuce, red cabbage, marrow
Fruit—watermelon, dried dates
Other—soft drink, confectionery, chocolate, manufactured baked goods, muffins, cakes, biscuits, donuts, sugar (most processed food has a high GI)

For a complete list of the GI of specific food go to glycemicindex.com.

GI, causing a large and rapid rise in blood sugar, while complex carbohydrates have a low GI and have a much smaller affect on blood sugar levels.

Recent studies have shown that eating low GI carbohydrates produces lower levels of circulating blood sugar. This results in more fat being used for energy, therefore helping you lose weight. Eating low GI carbohydrates also brings about lower levels of bad cholesterol (Low Density Lipoproteins) and higher levels of good cholesterol (High Density Lipoproteins). All the more reason to stay away from simple, refined high GI carbohydrates.

GEEK SPEAK

Glucoregulation is the maintenance of steady levels of glucose in the body; it is a vital part of homeostasis, and so keeps a constant internal environment around cells in the body. The hormone insulin is the primary regulatory factor in our body. It causes many tissue cells to take up glucose from circulation. It causes some cells to store glucose in the form of glycogen, and when stores are met it causes other cells to take it in and hold it as lipids (fat). Insulin also controls cellular electrolyte balances and amino acid uptake as well. Its absence turns off glucose uptake into cells, reverses electrolyte adjustments, begins glycogen breakdown and glucose release into the circulation by some cells, begins lipid release from lipid storage cells etc. The level of blood sugar is the most important signal to the insulin-producing cells. Because the level of circulatory glucose is largely determined by the intake of dietary carbohydrates, diet controls major aspects of metabolism via insulin. Since humans over-consume carbohydrates, especially low GI carbohydrates, it is not surprising Type 2 diabetes is epidemic. Another lifestyle disease that can be prevented and 90 per cent reversed through proper nutrition!

The glycemic index measures the rate at which a particular food/carbohydrate raises your blood sugar levels. Rated on a scale of 0 to 100:

* 0–55 = Low GI
* 56–69 = Medium GI
* 70+ = High GI.

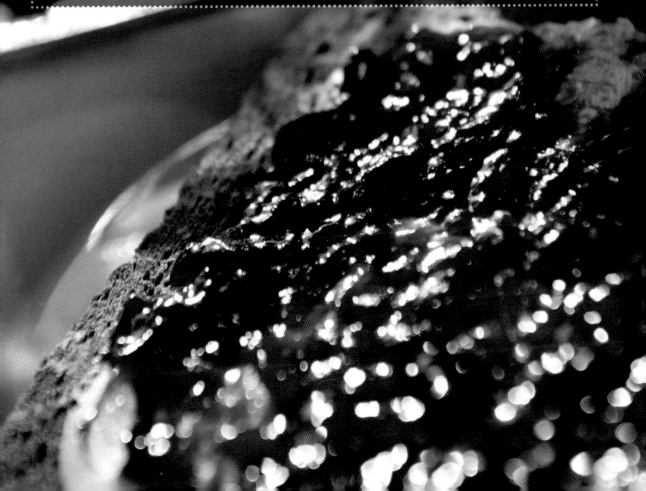

Whole grains have featured in the human diet since early civilisation. Once harvested, grains have a long shelf-life, providing energy during harsh seasons when fresh fruits and vegetables were scarce. Each region had their staple grains, for example, wheat in Australia, corn in America, and rice in Asia. Because of the active lifestyle and natural diet, very few people were overweight in those days.

Whole grains are an excellent source of nutrition, as they contain essential enzymes, iron, dietary fibre, vitamin E and B-complex vitamins.

Because they are low GI your body absorbs them slowly, providing sustained, high-quality energy.

Now we have access to many grains, so try them all and see which ones you like best. Cooked grains keep very well, so if you're busy cook enough for several meals and simply reheat with a little oil or water when you need. Also, roasting grains makes them more alkaline. Cooking larger grains like brown rice, barley and wheat berries (whole wheat kernels with the husk removed) in a pressure cooker speeds up cooking time and creates softer grains.

1 CUP OF GRAIN	WATER	COOKING TIME	CONTAINS GLUTEN?
Common Grains			
Brown rice	2 cups	45-60 minutes	no
Buckwheat (a.k.a. kasha)*	2 cups	20-30 minutes	no
Oats (whole groats)	3 cups	75-90 minutes	May have have traces
Oatmeal (rolled oats)	2 cups	20-30 minutes	May have have traces
Alternative Grains			
Amaranth**	3 cups	30 minutes	no
Barley (pearled)	2-3 cups	60 minutes	yes
Barley (hulled)	2-3 cups	90 minutes	yes
Bulgur (cracked wheat)	2 cups	20 minutes	yes
Cornmeal (a.k.a. polenta)	3 cups	20 minutes	no
Couscous*	1 cup	5 minutes	yes
Kamut	3 cups	90 minutes	yes
Millet	2 cups	30 minutes	no
Quinoa**	2 cups	15-20 minutes	no
Rye berries	3 cups	2 hours	yes
Spelt	3 cups	2 hours	yes
Wheat berries	3 cups	60 minutes	yes
Wild rice	4 cups	60 minutes	no

*Technically not a grain, but a small pasta product made from wheat that does not require soaking. Also note 1 cup of grain is enough for 2–4 people when cooked. ** **Is eaten as a grain but is actually a seed

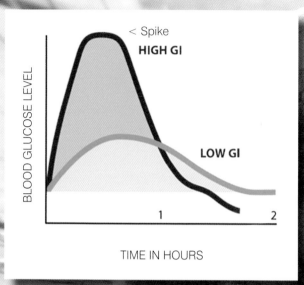

CARBS CAUSING AGEING

'Chronic inflammation lies at the root of virtually every disease process known to modern man—from weight gain, obesity and heart disease to autoimmune disorders like lupus, MS and rheumatoid arthritis.' - Dr. Chris Lydon, Yale University

There is plenty of research to support this statement, and now inflammation is the number one cause of ageing. I'm not talking about a swollen ankle inflammation, rather that inflammation that occurs at a cellular level inside your body.

Acute inflammation is your body's natural (and helpful) response to tissue damage. When you injure yourself your inflammatory response takes action. Before you know it, there is swelling, redness and a lot of heat around the injury. That's your body trying to heal and it's a positive thing. It throws in pain for good measure just so you don't get up and try to run a marathon when your body can't cope.

Chronic inflammation, also known as prolonged inflammation, is your body's destructive and negative response to excess environmental, physical and mental toxins from things like a poor diet, toxic chemicals exposure, anxiety and stress.

Eating sugar and other refined carbs cause a rapid increase in blood sugar and the following set of events in your body lead to inflammation of the cell.

We love our sugar. Over the last 50 years, we have more than doubled our consumption of sugar. We each now consume an average of 50 kg (110 lb) per year! That's about 22 teaspoons per day, which is over 450 calories or 1,890 kJ.

People in the Western world consume somewhere between 33kg (72.6lb) to 40kg (88lb) of sugar per year! Not only does sugar make us fat, it is rotting our teeth, it is a major cause of the type 2 diabetes epidemic, and it can even contribute to cancer. So why are we eating so much of this nasty white powder? Put simply, sugar is addictive.

Mike Adams, founder of naturalnews.com, doesn't sugar-coat his opinion of sugar:

'Refined white sugar is a pleasure drug. If you don't believe me, just put a spoonful on your tongue and observe the instantaneous effects. You'll experience a warming, comfortable feeling that makes you feel safe and happy. They're not called "comfort foods" by accident. Sugar is, essentially, a legalised recreational drug that is socially acceptable to consume. And yet, just like many other drugs, over time it destroys our health, rots our teeth, disrupts normal brain function, promotes heart disease and directly causes diabetes and obesity. The argument that "street drugs are outlawed because they're dangerous to a person's health" falls flat on its face when you consider what sugar does to the human body. It's a lot more dangerous than marijuana, for example, and yet marijuana is illegal to possess or consume.'

The effect sugar has on the brain is similar to pain-killing drugs such as morphine and heroin. Just like sugar, these drugs produce an almost instant feeling of calm and pleasure, making them addictive. Once food manufacturers understood this addictive effect, they began putting sugar in just about all processed food, from canned food, fruit juices and soft drinks to bread, breakfast cereals and 'health' bars. Even infant formula and baby food has added sugar. And now we are fatter and more addicted than ever.

Sugar qualifies as an addictive substance in two ways:

1. Eating a small amount creates a desire for more.
2. Quitting suddenly causes withdrawal symptoms such as headaches, mood swings, cravings and fatigue.

Aside from the physical addiction, many of us have also developed an emotional addiction to sugar. How many times as a child were you rewarded with a sweet treat? And when do you celebrate a special occasion with a bowl of fruit instead of a cake? If you're feeling down, a cup of spinach doesn't provide quite the same sympathetic hug as an ice cream, does it? But guess what, that sugar high is short-lived and you generally end up feeling worse. Sugar is a fattening, toxic substance, no matter how many pretty coloured sprinkles are used to disguise it.

HOW DID THIS HAPPEN?

If we go back to caveman times, studies show our DNA was wired to taste sweet or bitter to help us distinguish between food that was poisonous and food that was safe. Sweet mainly indicated safe. In addition, as humans cannot produce Vitamin C, we must get it from our food. And since Vitamin C is usually found in sweet foods, such as oranges, berries and plums, we can conclude that our natural desire for sweet things is our body's way of hunting foods rich in Vitamin C.

This wasn't a problem for our waistlines in hunter-gatherer times. But today, when we reach for a chocolate bar while we're sitting in front of a computer or TV, it's a very different story! So next time you have a sweet craving, opt for a handful of berries or a fresh orange juice—but not a manufactured one with 11 teaspoons of sugar!

Sugar is a simple carbohydrate that is found naturally in food such as grains, beans, vegetables and fruit. In its unprocessed state, sugar also contains a variety of vitamins, minerals and enzymes. When we eat brown rice or fruit, the natural carbohydrate is broken down steadily into separate glucose molecules. These molecules enter our bloodstream, where they are metabolised smoothly and evenly, allowing our body to absorb the nutrients without a big spike in blood sugar and the need for large doses of insulin. Nice, simple, and what our body knows.

However, refined, processed and simple sugar—usually extracted from sugar cane or beets, and known as sucrose (a.k.a. nasty drug)—has a totally different effect on our body. It lacks any nutrients (vitamins, minerals and fibre), so our body has to work a little harder to digest it. Metabolising the sucrose causes a depletion of minerals, enzymes and Vitamin B. It also pushes blood sugar levels sky-high, causing excitability and hyperactivity. Then insulin responds in a big way and our blood sugar drops to a low point, causing fatigue, weariness and depression. This roller-coaster effect is implicated in the onset of type 2 diabetes.

Just a little side note: stress depletes your body of Vitamin B. After a stressful day, on top of the stress you already have from your day, you may decide a sweet treat or glass of wine is in order—and we know alcohol is sugar. So you're not helping the situation, you're making it worse!

And if you think you're doing yourself a favour by cutting fat out of your diet—since fat has 9 calories or 37.7 kJ compared to sugar's 4 calories or 17 kJ—I'm about to rain on your parade again. It is sugar, not fat, that is making us fat!

Bring back omega-3s and get rid of sugar and watch how many ADHD children become normal kids! Good fats are an integral part of our diet and are generally accompanied by a host of vitamins and minerals our body needs.

Burning and storing fat is all about controlling your insulin levels. Eating refined sugar causes a spike in blood sugar, triggering a release of insulin, which leads to faster fat storage. In a healthy, slim person, 40 per cent of the sugar they eat is converted to fat. But in an overweight person, 60 per cent of the sugar they eat is converted to fat!

QUITTING COLD TURKEY

Sugar is a toxic substance that contributes nothing to your diet, except a lot of health issues. The best thing you can do is to quit eating it. But that's easier said than done.

To successfully quit, you need to know your main offenders, since food manufacturers sneak sugar into anything and everything and in various guises. Look for words ending in 'ose', such as sucrose, fructose, maltose, lactose, dextrose and maltodextrose.

Avoid syrups, especially high-fructose corn syrup (HFCS). This is very cheap, so is used in many processed foods, but according to a study conducted by the University of Pennsylvania, it boosts fat-storing and hunger hormones. It is found in many cereal bars, fruit drinks, tomato sauce, mayonnaise, pasta sauce and salad dressings.

Sugar may be listed on food labels as brown sugar, palm sugar, cane sugar, corn syrup, fructose, fruit juice concentrate, glucose (dextrose), high-fructose corn syrup, honey, invert sugar, lactose, maltose, molasses, raw sugar, table sugar (sucrose) or syrup. Read labels carefully and don't be surprised if you see sugar in three or four different varieties.

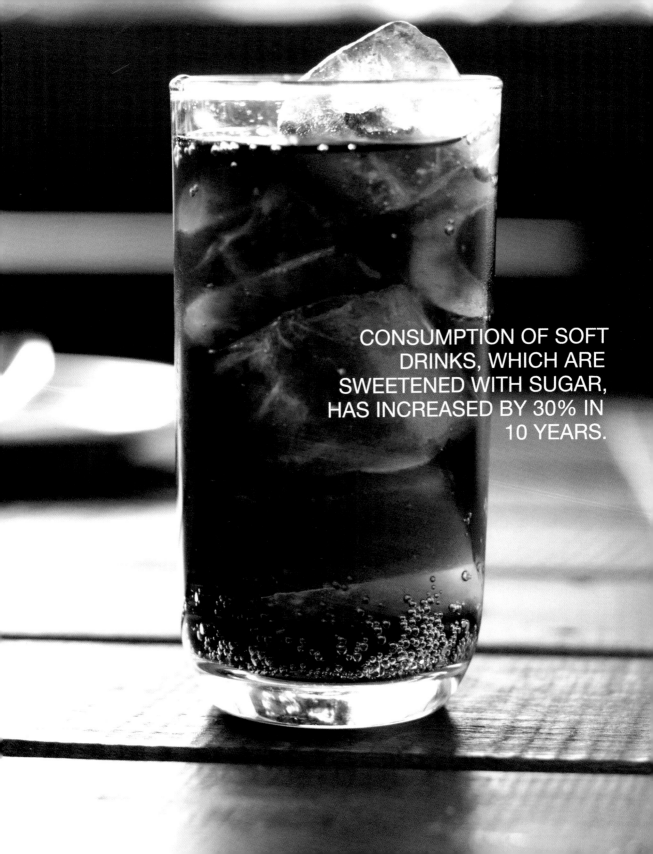

CONSUMPTION OF SOFT DRINKS, WHICH ARE SWEETENED WITH SUGAR, HAS INCREASED BY 30% IN 10 YEARS.

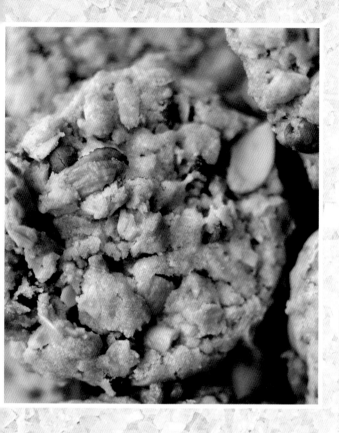

EFFECTS OF SUGAR

It is believed excessive consumption of sugar may play a role in the formation of many diseases, not just obesity and type 2 diabetes. Sugar:

* suppresses the immune system
* upsets your body's mineral balance
* contributes to hyperactivity, anxiety and depression
* contributes to a weakened defence against bacterial infection
* causes kidney damage
* increases the risk of coronary heart disease
* interferes with absorption of calcium and magnesium
* contributes to diabetes
* contributes to osteoporosis
* causes food allergies
* increases fluid retention.

HOW MUCH SUGAR IS HIDDEN IN OUR FOOD?

Food	Teaspoons of sugar
Special K (1½ oz/40 g serve)	1.5
Small tub of yoghurt (7 oz/200 g)	6*
Small fruit juice (15 fl oz/450 mL)	11

* Typically, the lower a yoghurt is in fat, the higher it is in sugar or artificial sweeteners. Steer clear.

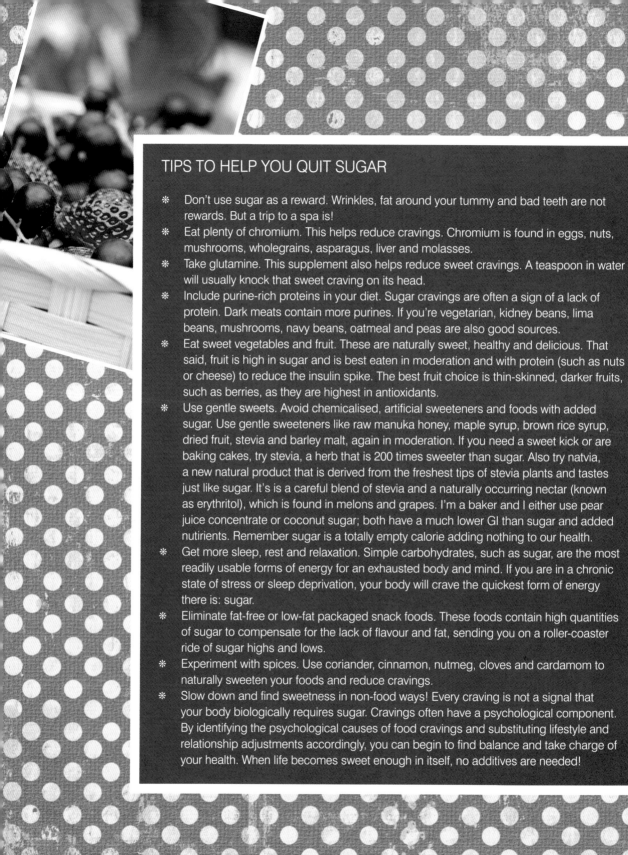

TIPS TO HELP YOU QUIT SUGAR

✳ Don't use sugar as a reward. Wrinkles, fat around your tummy and bad teeth are not rewards. But a trip to a spa is!

✳ Eat plenty of chromium. This helps reduce cravings. Chromium is found in eggs, nuts, mushrooms, wholegrains, asparagus, liver and molasses.

✳ Take glutamine. This supplement also helps reduce sweet cravings. A teaspoon in water will usually knock that sweet craving on its head.

✳ Include purine-rich proteins in your diet. Sugar cravings are often a sign of a lack of protein. Dark meats contain more purines. If you're vegetarian, kidney beans, lima beans, mushrooms, navy beans, oatmeal and peas are also good sources.

✳ Eat sweet vegetables and fruit. These are naturally sweet, healthy and delicious. That said, fruit is high in sugar and is best eaten in moderation and with protein (such as nuts or cheese) to reduce the insulin spike. The best fruit choice is thin-skinned, darker fruits, such as berries, as they are highest in antioxidants.

✳ Use gentle sweets. Avoid chemicalised, artificial sweeteners and foods with added sugar. Use gentle sweeteners like raw manuka honey, maple syrup, brown rice syrup, dried fruit, stevia and barley malt, again in moderation. If you need a sweet kick or are baking cakes, try stevia, a herb that is 200 times sweeter than sugar. Also try natvia, a new natural product that is derived from the freshest tips of stevia plants and tastes just like sugar. It's is a careful blend of stevia and a naturally occurring nectar (known as erythritol), which is found in melons and grapes. I'm a baker and I either use pear juice concentrate or coconut sugar; both have a much lower GI than sugar and added nutirients. Remember sugar is a totally empty calorie adding nothing to our health.

✳ Get more sleep, rest and relaxation. Simple carbohydrates, such as sugar, are the most readily usable forms of energy for an exhausted body and mind. If you are in a chronic state of stress or sleep deprivation, your body will crave the quickest form of energy there is: sugar.

✳ Eliminate fat-free or low-fat packaged snack foods. These foods contain high quantities of sugar to compensate for the lack of flavour and fat, sending you on a roller-coaster ride of sugar highs and lows.

✳ Experiment with spices. Use coriander, cinnamon, nutmeg, cloves and cardamom to naturally sweeten your foods and reduce cravings.

✳ Slow down and find sweetness in non-food ways! Every craving is not a signal that your body biologically requires sugar. Cravings often have a psychological component. By identifying the psychological causes of food cravings and substituting lifestyle and relationship adjustments accordingly, you can begin to find balance and take charge of your health. When life becomes sweet enough in itself, no additives are needed!

KEEPING IT CLEAN

Another recap—this time on carbohydrates. While you are on the Get Clean Get Lean program you do not want to go near high GI carbs, wheat or sugar. They are contraband for the next 28 days, although I bet you find life so good without them you probably won't go back!

Instead, you will get your sugar hit from fruit and sweet vegetables. And you'll get your energy from low GI carbs such as brown rice, oats, amaranth, millet, quinoa, buckwheat, plain rice cakes, spelt or rye bread, and starchy vegetables. Remember the portion plate? You only need about 25 per cent of your energy coming from carbs. Wondering how you'll cope without your cereal for breakfast? I guarantee you'll love eating real food to kick start your day.

When choosing bread—the heavier and darker the better. That light, sugar-filled, bleached, sliced white bread wrapped in plastic is soon to be a thing of the past. Once you've eaten proper wholegrain bread you won't be going back. If your bread is hard and stale within a day, then you know there are no preservatives in it. If it's still light and fluffy for a week ... hmmm!

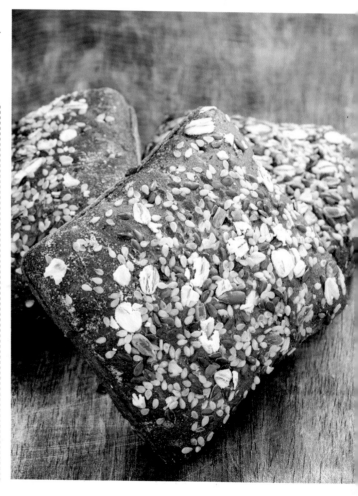

CLEAN CARBS

- While on the cleanse, avoid wheat and wheat-based products.

- Avoid all processed carbs, pasta, cakes, muffins, commercial breads etc.

- Under no circumstances should you have sugar!

- Most of your carbs will come from starchy vegetables while you are cleansing.

- Limit grains to a max. 1 serve/day. (1 serve = 1 oz/30 g) as they are low in the required detox nutrients and contribute to an acidic body.

- Try to eat organic and wholegrain foods.

- Only low GI carbs are allowed.

FATS

A healthy body needs some fat, which contains essential nutrients (that is, nutrients your body can't synthesise so you need to get them into your body through your diet). Your body uses dietary fat to make tissue and manufacture biochemicals, such as hormones. Fats in your diet are sources of energy that add flavour to food—puts the sizzle in the steak, so to speak. However, fats may also be hazardous to your health if you are eating the wrong kind in the wrong proportions; the trick is knowing the good from the bad. Unfortunately, as discussed in Carbohydrates, fats not only got tarred with the same brush in the 1980s and beyond, they also copped a bad rap. By now you understand that the right fats in the right amount are essential for good health. The chemical family name for fats and related compounds (such as cholesterol) is lipids. Liquid fats are called oils; solid fats are called, well, fat. With the exception of cholesterol, fats are high-energy nutrients. Gram for gram, fats have more than twice as much energy potential (calories) as protein and carbohydrates: 9 calories per fat gram versus 4 calories per gram for proteins and carbs.

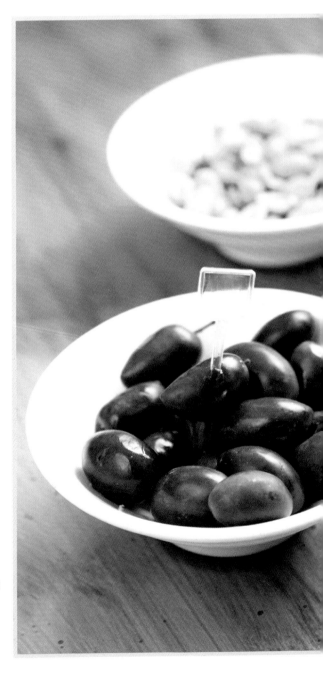

Some of the body fat made from food fat is visible. Even though your skin covers it, you can see the fat in the adipose (fatty) tissue in female breasts, hips, thighs, buttocks, and belly or male abdomen and shoulders. A little bit of this fat is actually OK as it:

* provides a source of stored energy
* gives shape to your body
* cushions your skin (imagine sitting for long times without your bum to pillow your bones)
* acts as an insulation blanket that reduces heat loss.

Other body fat is invisible. You can't see this body fat because it's tucked away in and around your internal organs.

CHOLESTEROL LEVELS INCREASE AS WE GET OLDER, PARTICULARLY AFTER MENOPAUSE IN WOMEN.

THE IMPORTANT ROLE OF HIDDEN FAT

Aside from the fat that you can squeeze at your waist or see on your body, there is fat deep within your body at a cellular level. Hidden fats are:

* part of every cell membrane (the outer skin that holds each cell together)

* a component of myelin, the fatty material that sheathes nerve cells and makes it possible for them to fire the electrical messages that enable you to think, see, speak, move, and perform the multitude of tasks natural to a living body. Brain tissue is also rich in fat.

* a shock absorber that protects your organs (as much as possible) if you fall or are injured

* a constituent of hormones and other biochemicals, such as vitamin D and bile. It's common knowledge that too much cholesterol and other fats can lead to disease, and that a healthy diet involves watching how much fatty food we eat. However, our bodies need a certain amount of fat to function—and we can't make it from scratch.

* Triglycerides, cholesterol and other essential fatty acids—the scientific term for fats the body can't make on its own—store energy, insulate us and protect our vital organs. They act as messengers, helping proteins do their jobs. They also start chemical reactions that help control growth, immune function, reproduction and other aspects of basic metabolism.

* The cycle of making, breaking, storing and mobilising fats is at the core of how humans and all animals regulate their energy. An imbalance in any step can result in disease, including heart disease and diabetes. For instance, having too many triglycerides in our bloodstream raises our risk of clogged arteries, which can lead to heart attack and stroke.

* Fats help the body stockpile certain nutrients as well. The fat-soluble vitamins—A, D, E and K—are stored in the liver and in fatty tissues.

POLY-UNSATURATED FAT

The body can synthesise many of the fats it needs for normal metabolism and good health. However, some essential components must be found from our diet, including the omega-3 (Ω-3) and omega-6 (Ω-6) polyunsaturated fatty acids.

Ω-3 fatty acids are unsaturated fatty acids and the most important nutritionally are: ∂-lipopenic acid, eicosapentaenoic acid (EPA) and docosahexaenoic acid (DHA). They are the immediate precursor of many eicosanoids, which control a number of important pathways highly relevant to ageing, including inflammation, immune function, clotting and cancer growth.

There is substantial evidence that a diet high in EPA and DHA can reduce the risk of heart disease and stroke, possibly by lowering blood pressure, improving blood triglyceride levels, stimulating local circulation and preventing clotting. These fats may also have beneficial effects on other problems associated with ageing, including varicose veins, arthritis, cognitive decline, Alzheimer's disease, depression, rheumatoid problems, as well as certain skin ailments. Research has also shown Ω-3 to be helpful in children with attention deficit hyperactivity disorder (ADHD).

It is recommended to eat a gram of EPA and DHA each day from animal fats, or 2–3 g per day of alpha-linolenic acid from seeds. This is equivalent to an oily fish meal 2 or 3 times a week.

Omega-6 fatty acids are a precursor for the synthesis of many regulatory eicosanoids. Ω-6 supports skin health, lowers cholesterol and helps make our blood 'sticky' so it can clot. However, when in excess, Ω-6 can lead to increased production of factors that favour inflammation, clotting and tissue injury, which can increase the risk of heart attack and stroke.

Linoleic acid is the most common dietary Ω-6 fat and is found in oils, eggs, cereals, grains, nuts and seeds. Evening primrose oil contains a high content of gamma-linolenic acid, another type of Ω-6 fatty acid.

Unfortunately, Ω-3 and Ω-6 compete for the same metabolic enzymes, so the Ω-6:Ω-3 ratio significantly influences the ratio of the ensuing eicosanoids (hormones), (e.g. prostaglandins, leukotrienes, thromboxanes, etc.) and alters the body's metabolic function. Research shows that the most promising health effects of essential fatty acids are achieved through a proper balance between Ω-6 and Ω-3. According to the experts, the lower the ratio the better. Best is 1:1, although up to 4:1 (omega 6: omega 3) is still very good.

. Most of us eating a Western diet have this ratio dangerously out of whack—around at best 10:1, however 20:1 is not uncommon.

Any imbalance can lead to a number of adverse consequences, including depression, heart attacks, stroke, arthritis, osteoporosis, inflammation and cancer. You can tip the balance in your favour and reduce these health risks by increasing your intake of Ω-3s. Equally important is the ability of Ω-3 to reduce the negative impact of excess consumption of Ω-6. By increasing Ω-3 in our diet, the risk of heart problems is reduced. Often the easiest way to do this is to take an Ω-3 supplement. Interestingly, over-consumption of Ω-6 fatty acids is the primary reason behind the need for Ω-3 supplementation.

Ratios of Ω-6 to Ω-3 fatty acids common oils:	
Flax	1:3
Canola	2:1
Olive	3-13:1
Soybean	7:1
Corn oil	46:1
Peanut & Sunflower	no Ω-3
Cotton & Grapeseed	almost no Ω-3

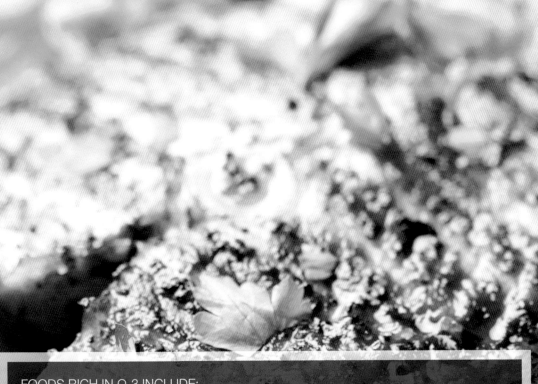

FOODS RICH IN Ω-3 INCLUDE:

- ✳ cold-water oily fish, such as salmon, herring, mackerel, anchovies, sardines and, to a lesser extent, tuna. (Farmed fish is higher in Ω-6 and lower in Ω-3 than fish from the sea.)

- ✳ meat from grass-eating animals, such as lamb or kangaroo. Organic, grass-fed beef has a Ω-6 to Ω-3 fat ratio of 2:1, compared to 4:1 or higher for grain-fed beef

- ✳ dairy products from grass-fed cows

- ✳ organic eggs (from chickens fed a diet of greens and insects, not battery hens fed on grain) or eggs from chickens fed flaxseeds (to fortify the egg with Ω-3s)

- ✳ a vegetarian diet can obtain significant amounts of Ω-3 fat from flaxseed (linseed), purslane, kiwifruit, lignon berries, black raspberries and walnuts

MONO-UNSATURATED FATS

Mono-unsaturated fats (MUFAs) are liquid at room temperature, but solid when refrigerated. They are also more resistant to going rancid than polyunsaturated fatty acids. The most common dietary MUFA is oleic acid, a Ω-9 fatty acid found in vegetable and seed oils, nuts, avocado and some meats. Most of these possibly beneficial compounds are destroyed by prolonged, high-temperature cooking or frying, so consider drizzling on your salad instead! A number of studies have suggested that a high intake of MUFAs, typical in most Mediterranean diets, can lower blood pressure, possibly by changing the composition of membrane lipids and proteins, or improving vascular function. Foods containing monounsaturated fats also lower LDL cholesterol.

SATURATED FATS

All natural products have a balance of saturated and unsaturated fats. Foods with a higher proportion of saturated fat include butter, coconut, nuts, dairy products (especially cream and cheese), chocolate, meat and eggs.

Increased intake of saturated fat from our diet contributes to heart disease, more because it raises bad (LDL) cholesterol than as a result of the dietary cholesterol itself. We should aim to reduce our intake of saturated fat to less than 7 per cent of our total calories by limiting our intake of dairy products, including whole milk, butter, cheese and ice cream. The meat of grass-fed animals and birds also contains much lower levels of saturated fat than conventional, grain-fed animals.

TRANS (THE NASTY) FATS

Most trans fats were deliberately created during the processing of vegetable oils (by hydrogenation) to make them solid at room temperature, to melt when baking (or eating) and more resistant to going off than animal fats like butter. Prolonged over-heating and deep-frying can also generate trans fats, which are transferred to the food.

Unlike other unsaturated fats, trans fats are toxic to a number of your important systems, contributing to heart disease, stroke, diabetes, obesity, insulin resistance, prostate cancer and infertility. In fact, trans fats increase the risk of heart disease more than any other component in your diet. Even a small intake is sufficient to start increasing your risk of heart disease. There appears to be no safe limit for trans fats. Avoid!

THE BAD AND THE GOOD (CHOLESTEROL)

Cholesterol is a lipid found in the membranes of every human cell, where it functions to keep our cell membranes flexible. It also has an important role in the production of bile, which is important for the digestion and absorption of fat, as well as fat-soluble vitamins such as Vitamins A, D, E and K. Cholesterol is also used in the body to synthesise Vitamin D, as well as a number of hormones important to the ageing process, such as cortisol, ostrogens and testosterone. Every day your body makes about 1 g of cholesterol and takes in another 20-30 per cent from food. Any food that contains animal fat also contains cholesterol, especially egg yolk, beef, pork, poultry and shrimp/prawns.

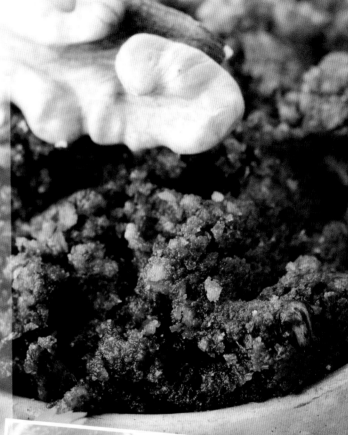

The body contains a number of different forms of cholesterol. The best known are Low Density Lipoprotein (LDL or bad cholesterol) and High Density Lipoprotein (HDL or good cholesterol). LDL cholesterol deposits in the walls of blood vessels, contributing to stiffening and narrowing, and ultimately their ageing. The higher your LDL cholesterol levels, the higher your risk of heart attack, stroke and other diseases of the blood vessels. On the plus side, for every one mmol/L that you increase or decrease your LDL cholesterol level with, your risk of death from cardiovascular disease changes by 20 per cent.

Another way to deal with the LDL problem is to offset it with HDL. HDL particles remove bad cholesterol from the walls of blood vessels and transport it back to the liver for excretion or safer storage sites (reverse cholesterol transport). People with high levels of HDL cholesterol have a lower risk of heart disease and stroke.

To give you an idea of how much fat to eat, here's a rough guide.

1 tbsp oil	20g
½ avocado	20g
1 oz/30 g almonds or walnuts	15g
1 egg	6g
7 oz/200 g low-fat yoghurt	4g

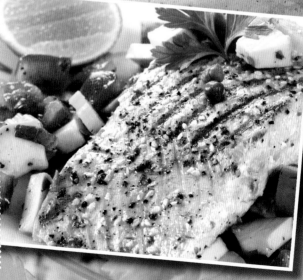

FATS IN A NUTSHELL

Just to recap, you need fat in your diet. Not only does it have vital health functions, it actually helps you stay fuller for longer. Being an advocate of all things natural, I would much rather you ate the real deal than the low-fat version. I'll go into this more when I introduce you to the Low HI way of eating. Seriously, if you have ever seen margarine being made and what colour it is before it is coloured to look like butter, I know you'd avoid it too. You can get plenty of great, natural plant-based fats to help maintain healthy cholesterol levels. Even a drizzle of olive oil is better than that stuff that comes in the plastic tub. The table below, supplied by the Institutue of Integrative Nutrition (IIN) summarises the main fats, where you'll find them, what they do and which ones to avoid ... did I mention to stay away from trans fats? Do!

SATURATED	MONOUNSATURATED	POLYUNSATURATED	TRANS FATTY ACID
Where you'll find them			
Beef, poultry, pork, cow's milk, coconut, avocado, palm oil, full-fat dairy	Avocados, olives, olive oil, nuts, sunflower oil, seeds, flathead, sablefish, mackerel, vegetables high in oleic-acid	Salmon, sardines, mackerel, herring, trout, fresh tuna, flax seed, pumpkin seeds, sesame seed, walnuts, flax seed oil, soybean oil	May be found in: margarine, processed foods, candy, chips, soda, flaky pastries, some peanut butters
What they are			
Solid at room temperature. Chemically, they consist of carbon atoms saturated with hydrogen atoms.	Liquid at room temperature, but become solid when chilled. Their chemical makeup consists of one double-bonded carbon molecule.	Liquid at room temperature and even when chilled. Their chemical makeup has more than one double-bonded carbon atom. Known as the 'omega fats'.	Most are created industrially by adding hydrogen bonds to liquid oils to make a more shelf-stable product. However, some trans fats occur naturally in beef, lamb butterfat and dairy.
Physiologic effects			
Potentially increase risk of heart disease.	Raise good HDL and lower LDL.	Raise good HDL and lower LDL. Omega-3 fatty acids are considered anti-inflammatory and are associated with lower risk of death.	Raise LDL and lower HDL, which leads to plaque build-up in arteries and increased risk of heart disease.
What to eat – What to avoid			
While opinions are mixed, it is generally recommended to limit consumption of red meats and butter.	Generally considered heart-healthy, these foods should be eaten daily.	Generally considered heart-healthy, strive to eat cold water fish three times per week and plant-based polyunsaturated oils often.	Entirely avoid products with partially-hydrogenated oils listed on the ingredients.

PLANT-BASED OILS

Best oils for salad
Always use cold-pressed and buy organic if possible.

* Extra virgin olive oil
* Flax seed oil (only eat raw, do not cook)
* Macadamia nut oil
* Raw coconut oil
* Avocado oil
* Hemp seed oil (only eat raw, do not cook)

Best oils for cooking
Use oils over medium heat and never let them smoke
as they can give off trans fats if heated too high.

* Raw coconut oil
* Macadamia nut oil
* Avocado oil
* Olive oil (low-medium temperatures only)

Use in moderation

* Grape seed oil
* Butter (great for pan-frying as it is very stable
  at high temperatures)
* Safflower, sunflower and palm oil (provided
  it's not hydrogenated)

Oils to avoid

* Peanut oil
* Canola oil
* Vegetable oil
* Soybean oil
* Margarine and anything oil that is
  hydrogenated

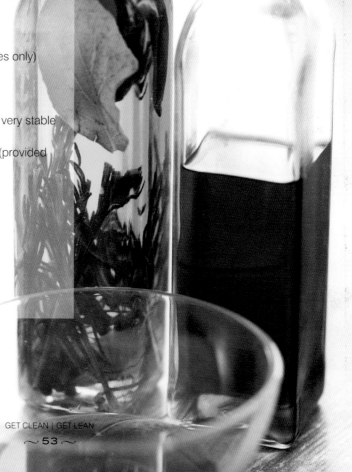

There is evidence to suggest that nut trees were grown as a source of human food as early as 10,000 BC, making them one of the earliest crops to be cultivated. Lately, however, nuts have been labelled as 'fattening' or, worse still, 'unhealthy'. I thought it was about time to dispel yet another diet myth and give you the real story on nuts.

Nuts contain high levels of protein. Protein in the diet is necessary for the growth, maintenance and repair of body tissue. Protein helps the building of cells, hormones and enzymes by providing the amino acids that form the 'building blocks' of life. Protein is also an important energy source for the body. Nuts have high levels of arginine (a type of protein), which helps our insulin work more effectively and contributes to the overall health of our blood vessels and consequently our cardiovascular system.

Protein is a thermogenic nutrient, which means it creates heat as it increases your metabolic rate and energy expenditure. Protein stimulates your metabolism much more than carbohydrate or fat, which is one of the reasons that high protein diets have become such a weight loss fad over the last five years. So nuts should NOT be avoided if you are on a diet (unless they are coated in chocolate).

NUTRIENTS IN NUTS

Almonds, pistachios, hazelnuts and brazil nuts are extremely high in calcium. Almonds are rich in some B vitamins and in minerals like potassium, zinc, calcium, magnesium and phosphorus. The Brazil nut is one of the richest vegetable sources of the antioxidant mineral selenium, which is very important for fertility and hormone metabolism. It also helps the thyroid gland to function.

A 1¾ oz/50 g serve of cashew nuts provides 20 per cent of a woman's daily iron requirement, while 20 fresh cashews provide a man's daily zinc requirement. Pistachio nuts have good amounts of iron and calcium, making them an excellent addition to the diet of vegetarians.

Peanuts and pistachios provide a good source of B vitamins, which are essential for energy production, protein metabolism and synthesis of red blood cells. Peanuts and hazelnuts are also high in vitamin E. Nuts are also a great source of fibre, which most people are not getting enough of in their diet.

There is no denying that nuts contain fat, but as you know, not all fats are created equal. Approximately 90 per cent of the fat in nuts is unsaturated (with a slight variation depending on the type of nut). Unsaturated fats have now been proven to be essential for the health of your heart and cell membranes, among other things we've covered.

Nuts have a low GI so they don't cause a rapid fluctuation in blood sugar like some snacks you might have relied on in the past. They tend to satisfy hunger and cravings for longer.

Just one small handful (1 oz/30 g) of nuts (about five walnuts) every day will not only get you through the snack-attack stage, but also help boost your immune system and lower your blood cholesterol levels. Nuts may help reduce the risk of heart disease and other diseases of ageing, and may also help prevent osteoporosis.

Provided your nut of choice is raw (organic if possible) and unsalted, nuts are a great option for your energy, fibre, fat and protein requirements.

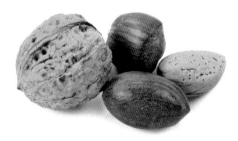

IT'S OK TO GO NUTS

* Energy controlled diets that include nuts result in greater weight loss than those that don't.

* Tree nuts include almonds, Brazil nuts, cashews, chestnuts, hazelnuts, macadamias, pecans, pine nuts, pistachios and walnuts.

* On average, adults need to increase their consumption of nuts by 350 per cent to meet the recommended handful (1 oz/30g) of nuts.

* Nuts help to suppress your appetite and keep you feeling satisfied in two ways: their high protein and fibre content helps to keep you feeling full for longer and nuts also release satiety hormones (such as cholecystokinin CCK) in the digestive system.

* Kick start your metabolism with a handful of nuts. A review of intervention trials found metabolism increases after eating nuts.

* If you swap a 1¾ oz/50 g bag of potato crisps for 1¾ oz/50 g nuts (around two handfuls) the nuts provide three times more protein, with nearly half the saturated fat and a fraction of the sodium, twice the fibre, vitamin E and a range of minerals: magnesium, calcium, iron, zinc, copper, manganese and selenium.

* Did you know? Nut eaters tend to weigh less than people who avoid nuts.

* If you chew nuts less you'll absorb less fat. Similarly if you eat whole nuts instead of nut butters less fat is absorbed.

* A handful of nuts (1 oz/30 g) at least five times a week can reduce your risk of developing heart disease by 30–50 per cent.

COCONUTS

Coconut is another one of those nuts that has copped a bad rap due to its fat content. Technically coconut is drupe—almost a cross between a fruit, nut and seed. You can see where this is going can't you? Nut, seed and fruit in a tight, husky packet ... that's one uber health food! So, why all the bad press on something that has so many benefits? Mainly because the oil extracted from the meat of mature coconuts is primarily saturated fat.

Now, here's the thing, these fats are plant-based saturated fats, meaning the coconut fat is composed predominately of medium-chain fatty acids (MCFAs). The physiological effects of MCFA are distinctly different from the long-chain fatty acids, which are found in animal-based saturated fats. Since MCFA fats are small enough to be absorbed into the cells where they're quickly converted to energy, they are less likely to be stored as fat. And there is ample research that shows people lose more weight (or fat) when they include a teaspoon or two of coconut oil in their diet.

A recent study by the Garvan Institute of Medical Research found that coconut oil protects against insulin resistance, reducing the risk of type 2 diabetes. It is this process that not only reduces the amount of fat we store, but improves insulin sensitivity.

Coconut oil (and milk, cream and flesh):

* protects against heart disease by increasing good cholesterol and lowering the ratio of bad and good cholesterol
* helps treat malnutrition because it is easy to digest and absorb
* kills disease-causing bacteria, fungi, yeasts and viruses because of the antimicrobial effects of its MCFA (mainly due to lauric acid)
* helps to prevent strokes and brain disorders such as Alzheimer's and Parkinson's
* boosts metabolism and increases energy because it is more likely to be burned as fuel than stored as body fat
* provides a good source of fibre (when the flesh is eaten).

Because the oil from coonuts is saturated, it means it is stable at high temperatures (like butter), so it is the ideal oil to cook with, especially when making Asian stir-frys.

If you haven't heard all the buzz about coconut water (specifically the water from the young coconut) you must have been hiding under a rock. The cloudy water is packed with electrolytes and minerals to replenish hydration levels within the body, making it a much better choice for rehydration than sugary, commercial electrolyte drinks. It also contains a great array of vitamins and minerals including B-complex vitamins such as riboflavin, niacin, thiamin, pyridoxine and folates. And it is rich in bioactive enzymes that help aid digestion and metabolism.

No wonder they call the coconut tree the Tree of Life!

KEEPING IT CLEAN

F ats are interesting, as many people avoid them especially if they are trying to lose weight. Hopefully by now you realise that fats are vital and can assist with weight loss if the right amount and the right fats are eaten. There is ample research to show that people who eat nuts lose more weight than people who don't while on a weight loss program. And cold-pressed coconut oil (although it has an amount of saturated fats) is super for your overall health. It's a great cooking medium, like olive oil, as it doesn't denature and give off trans fats at high temperatures like most oils.

While you are on the cleanse, reduce or even avoid animal fats if you can. Stick to raw and organic where possible and use cold-pressed oils. You'll get plenty of the good fats from nuts, seeds, avocados, olives and the odd egg or piece of fish.

HOW MUCH FAT?

30 per cent of your total kilojoules (calories) consumed should come from fat. This translates to:

* 2 oz/55 g/day for an adult moderately-active woman who's consuming 8400 kJ / 2000 calories a day
* 3 oz/85 g/day for an adult moderately-active man who's not on a diet (10 500 kJ/2500 calories)
* 1½ oz/40 g/day for an adult female who wants weight loss (5000 kJ/1200 calories)

Remember this is for total fat. You should also think about the type and quality of the fat – put the emphasis on mono- and polyunsaturated fats in preference to saturated fats, unless MCFAs. And void trans fats at all costs!

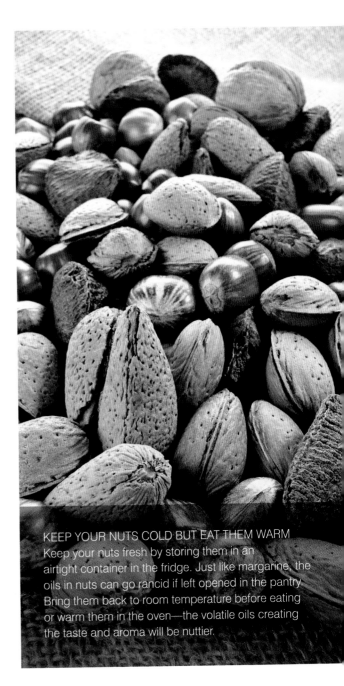

KEEP YOUR NUTS COLD BUT EAT THEM WARM
Keep your nuts fresh by storing them in an airtight container in the fridge. Just like margarine, the oils in nuts can go rancid if left opened in the pantry. Bring them back to room temperature before eating or warm them in the oven—the volatile oils creating the taste and aroma will be nuttier.

DAIRY

Dairy foods are all the products that come from the milk of animals, mainly cows, sheep and goats. Milk, butter, cream, cheese, yoghurt and ice-cream are the main dairy products we consume in the Western diet. Even though there are health benefits of diary foods (high in calcium, potassium, protein and Vitamins A, D, E and K) there is also a lot of not-so-nice things about dairy.

Firstly, there is a school of thought that says humans are only meant to drink milk for the first few years of their life. Milk is highly specific, containing hormones and nutrients designed for the various stages of life. For example, colostrum is jam-packed with fats, antibodies, vitamins and minerals to help a newborn cope with the first few days of life and exposure to everything outside of the safe haven of the womb. Once we have been weaned, about 75 per cent of people (25 per cent of Caucasians and 80 per cent of Asians, Native Americans or African origin) stop producing lactase, the enzyme needed to digest the milk sugar, lactose.

Humans are the only mammals who, once weaned from their mother's milk, continue to drink milk. Not only do we continue to drink milk, it is the milk from other mammals. Is this the best thing for us to be doing in regards to our health? Research is for and against this theory. However, the amount of people with lactose intolerance—the most common allergy—says a lot.

Over half the world's population survives and thrives without dairy food. In fact, you can get calcium from many other sources (seeds, nuts and beans) without having to rely on dairy products. Also, dairy products have also been linked to an increase in breast, prostate and colo-rectal cancer.

Here is an interesting fact about dairy: some people have an immediate allergic reaction to milk and this is detected by increased levels of the antibody immunoglobulin E (IgE). Some people have a more delayed reaction, which is identified with the presence of the antibody immunoglobulin G (IgG). (If you recall, we discussed this when we spoke of intolerance to gluten, the protein in wheat.) The protein in milk that causes a similar response is casein. And what I find even more interesting, milk from animals (other than our mother) is, like wheat, a relatively new addition to the human diet.

Unfortunately, casein does find its way into many foods from bread and cereals to packaged food, including crisps.

While you are on the Get Clean Get Lean program, I recommended you avoid dairy food. If you can't, then try eating goat's cheese and yoghurt. Goat's milk tends to be less exposed to all the hormones pumped into cows and sheep to get them to produce more milk, and it is closest to human milk in molecular structure. Most of us have a big enough struggle controlling our own hormones let alone those from another mammal. After you have completed the program and you start adopting the Low HI way of eating, if you do have to have dairy, please go for the real deal. Diet yoghurts make me shaky just thinking about their sugar content. Full cream milk is only 4 per cent fat, so if it was advertised as 96 per cent fat-free it would have a better image. Once you remove the fat, you also take away the fat-soluble vitamins.

For all the milkshake lovers and hot chocolate connoisseurs out there, there are plenty of milk alternatives, with less saturated fat and more goodness, such as almond, rice and coconut milk. Seriously, you can survive without dairy, just try swapping milk for a nut or rice milk and see how you feel.

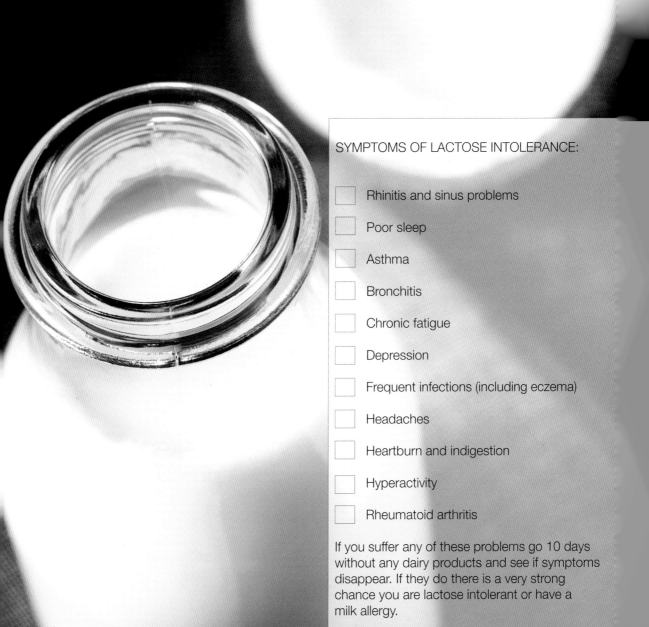

SYMPTOMS OF LACTOSE INTOLERANCE:

- [ ] Rhinitis and sinus problems
- [ ] Poor sleep
- [ ] Asthma
- [ ] Bronchitis
- [ ] Chronic fatigue
- [ ] Depression
- [ ] Frequent infections (including eczema)
- [ ] Headaches
- [ ] Heartburn and indigestion
- [ ] Hyperactivity
- [ ] Rheumatoid arthritis

If you suffer any of these problems go 10 days without any dairy products and see if symptoms disappear. If they do there is a very strong chance you are lactose intolerant or have a milk allergy.

FIBRE

Although fibre could fall under the Carbohydrate section, it is worth a special mention. Since there are so many processed foods in our diet, many of us aren't getting enough of this vital nutrient. Dietary fibre is found in cereals, seeds, nuts, fruits and vegetables and is the indigestible parts of plants, which pass relatively unchanged through our stomach and intestines. The main role of fibre is to keep the digestive system healthy and you regular.

It also contributes to other processes, such as stabilising glucose and cholesterol levels. In countries with traditionally high-fibre diets, diseases such as bowel cancer, diabetes and coronary heart disease are much less common than in Western countries.

Most people do not consume enough fibre. On average, people consume 20–25 g of fibre daily. The Heart Foundation recommends that adults should aim to consume approximately 25–30 g daily.

TYPES OF FIBRE

There are two main categories of fibre (although I have snuck in a third). They are beneficial to the body and most plant foods contain a mixture of both types. They are:

Soluble fibre—includes pectins, gums and mucilage, which are found mainly in plant cells. One of its major roles is to lower LDL (bad) cholesterol levels. When blood cholesterol levels are high, fatty streaks and plaques are deposited along the walls of arteries. This can make them dangerously narrow and lead to an increased risk of coronary heart disease. It is thought that soluble fibre lowers blood cholesterol by binding bile acids (which are made from cholesterol to digest dietary fats) and then excreting them.

Good sources of soluble fibre include fruits, vegetables, oat bran, barley, seed husks, flaxseed, psyllium, dried beans, lentils, peas, dates, soy milk and soy products. Soluble fibre can also help prevent constipation.

Insoluble fibre—includes cellulose, hemicelluloses and lignin, which make up the structural parts of plant cell walls. A major role of insoluble fibre is to add bulk to faeces and to prevent constipation and associated problems such as haemorrhoids. Good sources include wheat bran, corn bran, rice bran, the skins of fruits and vegetables, nuts, seeds, dried beans and wholegrain foods.

Resistant starch—while not traditionally thought of as fibre, it acts in a similar way. Resistant starch is the part of starchy food (approximately 10 per cent) that resists normal digestion in the small intestine. It is found in many unprocessed cereals and grains, unripe bananas, potatoes and lentils, and is added to bread and breakfast cereals as Hi-Maize. It can also be formed by cooking and manufacturing processes such as snap freezing.

Resistant starch is also important in bowel health. Bacteria in the large bowel ferment and change the resistant starch into short-chain fatty acids, which are important to bowel health and may protect against cancer. These fatty acids are also absorbed into the bloodstream and may play a role in lowering blood cholesterol levels.

DRINK LOTS OF WATER

Not only does water keep you hydrated, it keeps things moving. A high-fibre diet doesn't prevent or cure constipation unless you drink water. If your diet is high in fibre, please drink water, otherwise you'll suffer abdominal discomfort or constipation.

KEEPING THE DIGESTIVE TRACT HEALTHY & YOUR WEIGHT DOWN

The principal advantage of a diet high in fibre is improving the health of the digestive system. The digestive system is lined with muscles that massages food along the gastrointestinal (GI) tract from the first mouthful until the eventual waste is passed out of the bowel. This series of muscle contractions is called peristalsis. Since fibre is relatively indigestible, it adds bulk to the faeces.

In the GI tract, soluble fibre soaks up water like a sponge, which helps to bulk out the faeces and allows it to pass through the gut more easily. It acts to slow down the rate of digestion. This slowing down effect is usually overridden by insoluble fibre, which does not absorb water and speeds up the time that food passes through the gut.

Since fibrous foods are often bulky they are quite filling. Soluble fibre forms a gel that slows down the emptying of the stomach and the transit time of food through the digestive system. This makes you feel fuller for longer. It also delays the absorption of sugars from the intestines. This helps to maintain lower blood sugar levels and prevent a rapid rise in blood insulin levels, which has been linked with obesity and an increased risk of diabetes (as we've discussed).

For this reason, fibrous foods (which generally have a low GI) are great to help you maintain a healthy weight, lose weight and stop insulin surges.So, even though it's not the most exciting topic in the food story, it is a valuable one.

During the Get Clean Get Lean program you will be getting a lot of fibre, primarily from veggies, beans, legumes, nuts, seeds and some fruit. You'll definitely hit the 1 oz/30 g daily mark, which is why it's super important you keep up your water intake.

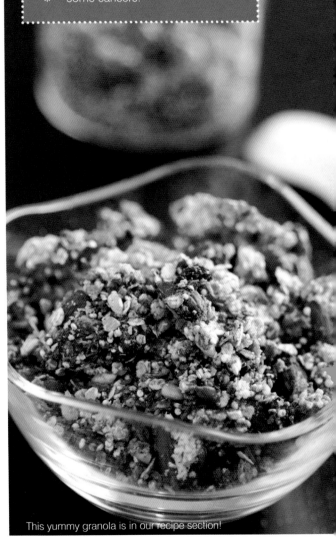

DISORDERS THAT CAN ARISE FROM A LOW-FIBRE DIET INCLUDE:
* constipation
* irritable bowel syndrome
* diverticulitis
* heart disease
* some cancers.

This yummy granola is in our recipe section!

ANTIOXIDANTS

The oxygen we breathe is an amazing substance. When combined at a cellular level with the food we eat, its unique reactivity provides you with the energy needed to fuel your movements and sustain many functions vital for life.

Ah, but oxygen is a double-edged sword! This same reactivity leads to production of highly damaging free radicals in our cells. Free radicals have been proven to play a major role in the process of ageing and degenerative diseases. These free radicals are toxic, and the very thing you will be mopping up and reducing during your Get Clean Get Lean program.

However, while oxygen is essential for life, the consequences of harnessing it to produce energy ultimately contributes to our demise!

When you add to this process the ravages of stress, heavy exercise, sun, pollution and other environmental factors, it sounds like we're all going down with the sinking ship.

But all is not lost, as there are also these wonderful things called antioxidants. I'm sure you've heard the word before, but maybe you aren't quite sure what they are or what they actually do. I can guarantee, by the end of this Get Clean program they will be your best friends. Antioxidants act like guards for all the cells in your body, helping stave off the early phases of ageing and protecting our immune system.

There is currently a great deal of interest in how free radical damage and antioxidants affect the ageing process. Jeff Coombes, Associate Professor in the School of Human Movement Studies at the University of Queensland, says, 'There is increasing evidence that many degenerative diseases, such as cancer, cardiovascular disease, immune-system decline, brain dysfunction and cataracts, may also be linked to free radical damage. Evidence that some of this damage can be decreased by antioxidants has led to increased research and increased use of nutritional antioxidants, with the goals of slowing the ageing process and protecting against degenerative diseases.'

Antioxidants are either:

1. **exogenous**—obtained from our diet or supplements, including Vitamins A, C and E
2. **endogenous**—made within our body.

Exogenous antioxidants are compounds (phytochemicals) found in brightly coloured fruits and vegetables. We have known for some time that these play an important role in protecting the body. However, little is spoken of the critical role played by endogenous antioxidants, which are also potent in preventing free radical damage. The five key endogenous antioxidants are:

1. superoxide dismutase (SOD), which plays a critical role in neutralising the most potent free radicals
2. catalase
3. glutathione peroxidase (Gpx)
4. alpha lipoic acid (ALA)
5. coenzyme Q10 (CoQ10).

Research has found that boosting cellular levels of endogenous antioxidants with supplements can help stave off age-related diseases, including cancer, heart disease, diabetes and Alzheimer's. Over 80 scientific studies have found that bioactive polysaccharides (enzymes) increase our body's production of the three most important endogenous antioxidants—SOD, catalase and Gpx. These potent enzymes are systemic, reaching every cell in your body, not just the gastrointestinal tract, so their effect is far-reaching. Elements found in certain natural foods, such as the bioactive polysaccharides in the Goji berry, help protect our endogenous antioxidants, such Glutathione (Gpx) is produced by every cell in your body and the primary protector and detoxifier of the cell. It is also the cell's first line of defence against the attack of free radicals, chemical toxins, radiation and heavy metals.

According to Dr David Katz, Director of Yale University's Prevention Research Centre, 'It is really the most important antioxidant. It's the one the body relies on to clean up critical toxins. If you're chronically run down; if you're chronically fatigued; if your body just isn't firing on all cylinders, low glutathione may be part of it, both cause and effect.' This view is backed up by Dr Oz; he says 'it is the most powerful antioxidant you've never heard of!' The reason you may not of heard of it is because your body produces it, however it is one of the most researched molecules (more so than Vitamin C) and under-estimated antioxidants.

So what is the best strategy for boosting your antioxidant protection? Well, the evidence suggests that, rather than large single doses of antioxidant supplements (eg. Vitamins A, C, E and the mineral selenium), it may be better to use low-dose synergistic combinations of these nutrients.

This should not be at the expense of harnessing the antioxidant power of phytochemical-rich fruits, especially berries, vegetables and other antioxidant-rich foods. As a rule of thumb, the darker and more vivid the colour of the food, the higher the antioxidant capacity. So for example, dark red cabbage is higher in antioxidant capacity than green cabbage, which in turn is higher in antioxidant capacity than white cabbage.

I try to get all my nutrients from food as I'm not a great tablet taker, however there are a couple of supplements I swear by, mainly because I exercise a lot, live in the city and I am constantly in a race with the clock (a self-denial way of saying I am exposed to stress). Plus, I have done a DNA test that shows I have a variation on one of the major genes associated with the detoxification process (meaning my liver is not an optimum detoxer). The antioxidant I take is a product called Cellgevity™, which is a potent supplement that is packed full of the five key endogenous antioxidants. It also has the unique ability to work at a cellular level stimulating your cells to produce Gpx. So technically, your body is producing the glutathione, however you're just giving it a little help. Your cell's ability to produce this antioxidant declines with age, as well as, stress, large toxic load, poor diet and lifestyle etc. So I highly recommend this regardless of whether you are doing the Get Clean program or not.*

PEOPLE WITH HIGHER GLUTATHIONE LEVELS HAVE:

- [ ] less inflammation
- [ ] reduced joint discomfort
- [ ] strengthened immune system
- [ ] more energy
- [ ] improved stamina and endurance
- [ ] faster recovery from exercise
- [ ] greater mental clarityand focus
- [ ] better sleep.

*Cellgevity™ is avaialble from krisabbey.com

THE ORAC SCALE

There is now a much more scientific method of estimating antioxidant capacity of food. This method is based on Oxygen Radical Absorbance Capacity (ORAC) and uses values derived from laboratory experiments. The higher the ORAC value, the better the food will be at deactivating the damaging, oxygen-free radicals (see table).

The best advice is to consume a wide range of high ORAC foods each day. 'It may be that combinations of nutrients found in foods have greater protective effects than each food nutrient taken alone,' says Guohua (Howard) Cao, a physician and chemist who developed the ORAC assay. You may have heard of the phrase 'Eat A Rainbow'? That simply means eat a food with a lot of different colours—and no, not of the artificial kind. Think big, bright, fresh colourful salads.

The use of ORAC values to rate the antioxidant capacity of foods is not yet widespread, but you can bet your bottom dollar that it will become much more popular soon. In the US, the FDA already recommends a daily ORAC intake of 7000 units per day to maintain optimum health and to help your body fight free radicals and diseases like cancer and heart disease. If you have high exposure to toxins, exercise a lot or are constantly faced with stress, you will need to increase this amount to about 9000.

FOOD	ORAC units per 3½ oz/ 100 g
Goji berries	25,300
70% cocoa dark chocolate	13,500
Pomegranate	10,500
Prunes	5,770
Apples (red delicious)	4,270
Raisins	2,830
Blueberries	2,400
Garlic	2,320
Blackberries	2,040
Spinach	1,700

Sources: US Dept of Agriculture; Brunswick Laboratories; Journal of American Chemical Society

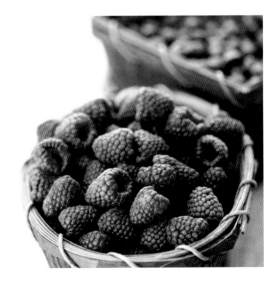

GEEK SPEAK

Phytochemicals are often responsible for giving a plant its characteristic colours and flavours. Many of these compounds display remarkable antioxidant capacities—tens or even hundreds of times greater than the antioxidant nutrients. Examples include the carotenoid family found in red and green fruits and vegetables, the flavonoid family found in citrus fruits, the tocotrienol family found in nuts, seeds and wheatgerm, and a number of sulphur-containing compounds, such as sulphorane, found in broccoli, and allicin, found in garlic. As a general rule of thumb, the deeper and more vivid the colour of the fruit or vegetable, the higher the phytochemical content and therefore its antioxidant activity.

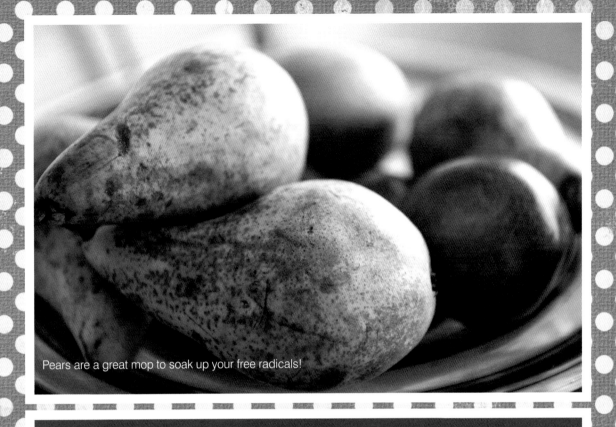

Pears are a great mop to soak up your free radicals!

WHAT ARE FREE RADICALS?

Free radicals are transient, but extremely reactive, chemicals. The production of free radicals unavoidably occurs in your body during the metabolism of fats, proteins and carbohydrates. When these nutrients are combined with oxygen to produce energy (aerobic metabolism) the by-product is a toxic free radical. They are sometimes called 'Reactive Oxygen Species' (ROS) or 'oxygen radicals'. Let's stick to calling them free radicals!

Although your cells have a very good antioxidant defence systems to quench and neutralise harmful free radicals (those endogenous antioxidants), however these defence systems are not 100 per cent efficient and, over time, biochemical damage gradually accumulates, leading to a reduction in cellular function. This means your ability to fight (or mop up) these free radicals declines as we age. And as stated many times previously, poor diet, too much processed food, stress and toxic exposure all put pressure on your body's ability to detoxify. Which is why it is important to give you body a break and do a cleanse from time to time. Most scientists now believe that accumulated cellular free radical damage lies at the heart of the ageing process and many degenerative diseases such as cancer, autoimmune diseases and Alzheimer's.

Because oxygen fuels exercise, sportspeople process and use larger volumes of oxygen and at faster rates than the majority of the population, so they may benefit from higher intakes of antioxidant nutrients to bolster their defences. So if you are a keen exerciser, all the more reason to eat a rainbow and possibly take a supplement.

CHOCOLATE: WHY DO WE LOVE IT?

The act of giving chocolates to loved ones on Valentine's Day began in the 1800s as a romantic gesture, perhaps because chocolate contains phenylethylamine, a natural chemical that acts on the brain to mimic the happy feeling of being in love.

Chocolate is not an addictive food, although if you love and crave chocolate you obviously believe otherwise! Chocolate is full of mood-enhancing chemicals. It contains the same mood-enhancing chemical found in marijuana, albeit in very small quantities. What we crave more than the nutrients in chocolate is this sensory experience and its association with happy times and special occasions. Chocolate also contains fat, which in itself satisfies hunger. The key ingredient of chocolate is cocoa, providing that rich, distinctive flavour. Cocoa beans grow in large pods on cacao trees in tropical rain forests. After the pods are picked from the trees, the cocoa beans are fermented in the sun, where the natural sugars combine with the heat and oxygen to develop their distinctive flavour. After fermentation, the beans are dried, packed and sold for processing.

During processing, the cocoa beans are heated and the centre of the bean is extracted and ground to produce chocolate liquor. This is exposed to varying degrees of pressure and temperature to produce either liquid cocoa butter or solid cakes of cocoa powder. Different combinations of cocoa butter and cocoa powder produce different types of chocolate products. Sweet-eating chocolate is a combination of unsweetened cocoa, sugar, cocoa butter and perhaps a little vanilla. Milk chocolate has milk added and contains less unsweetened cocoa.

For many years, in an effort to make great tasting chocolate, manufacturers removed the bitter flavours or masked it with sugar, but they soon discovered that these bitter flavours were in fact antioxidants called polyphenols. So a good rule of thumb, the darker the chocolate the better it is, or at least the higher its antioxidant value.

Current research findings suggest that liquid or dry cocoa extracts can be included in foods, food supplements and pharmaceuticals due to the stated health benefits. However, the processing of raw cocoa beans can result in a degradation of the valuable phenolic components that act as antioxidants. There are a number of great raw chocolate brands around and there is also the home-made chocolate recipe in this book, which is raw and delicious. And it is fine to eat in small amounts on the Get Clean program—a small amount—provided it is dark, preferably raw and doesn't have added sugar (you'll get used to the bitter taste if you're not already).

DID YOU KNOW?

* St Valentine was a priest who continued to perform secret marriages for Roman soldiers and their sweet-hearts who Emperor Claudius II had forbidden to marry. When found out, he was beheaded on 14 February 269 AD and is now the Patron Saint of Lovers.
* In the early 1500s, the Aztecs drank xocoatl (pronounced shocolatle) made from cocoa beans of the cacao tree, honey, spices and vanilla. It was believed to have special health properties and was drunk as a restorative and aphrodisiac. Cocoa beans were valuable as they were also used as currency. In 1753, cacao trees were given the classification name *Theobroma cacao*, which is Greek for 'Food of the Gods'.

While we are still on the subject of antioxidants, chocolate and wine both have high levels of antioxidants. They both fall within the category of 'I know I shouldn't, but I have heard they are healthy, so it's OK to indulge!'

OK, I'm about to share some really, really good news. The cocoa bean, which we use to make chocolate, is one of the healthiest foods on the planet. It's only when we add sugar, hydrogenated fats and sickly, goey centres to it that we undo all of this humble bean's goodness.

The main factor giving rise to claims that chocolate is good for you is the discovery that cacao contains natural antioxidants called procyanidins, from the antioxidant group called flavonoids. These have been shown to be more stable than the antioxidants found in green tea and wine and have a stronger effect in the body. Procyanidins have also been shown to be effective in relaxing some of the blood vessels in the body, which may benefit the heart.

In one study, people eating dark chocolate and cocoa powder were found to have increased levels of antioxidants. This prevented 'bad' cholesterol (LDL) in their blood from being oxidised, so it is unable to harden their arteries. Their levels of 'good' cholesterol (HDL) also went up. These antioxidants may also stop the blood from becoming too 'sticky', so there is less pressure on the heart to pump blood through your body.

Research is currently under way to determine if chocolate can prevent age-related high blood pressure. This theory was developed when it was discovered that an indigenous island-dwelling group in Central America called the Kuna Amerinds do not experience typical age-related increases in blood pressure. Apart from a diet consisting of locally grown fruit and vegetables like bananas, plantains (from the banana family), yucca (a starchy tuber), yams, corn, mangoes and fish, they also consume an average of five cups per day of a cocoa beverage that is high in flavanoids. I should probably stress here that the cocoa was from naturally dried beans, not the instant drinking chocolate that comes in a box laden with sugar! There is a lot of research currently underway on the benefits of cocoa—so watch this space.

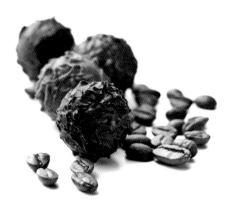

Research has shown that cacao is rich in flavanoids. Benefits include:

* promotion of cardiovascular health
* decreased oxidation of LDL to prevent atherosclerosis or plaque formation
* reduction in LDL cholesterol
* elevation in HDL cholesterol
* suppression of decay-causing bacteria and plaque formation (Water-soluble cocoa extracts)
* antidepressant and euphoric effects (from tryptophan in chocolate)
* stimulant effects (theobromine, phenylethylamine)
* increases the antioxidant level of the blood
* prevents blood fats from oxidising or getting sticky
* reduces the blood's ability to clot and increases the dilation or elasticity of blood vessels, thus reducing the risk of heart disease.

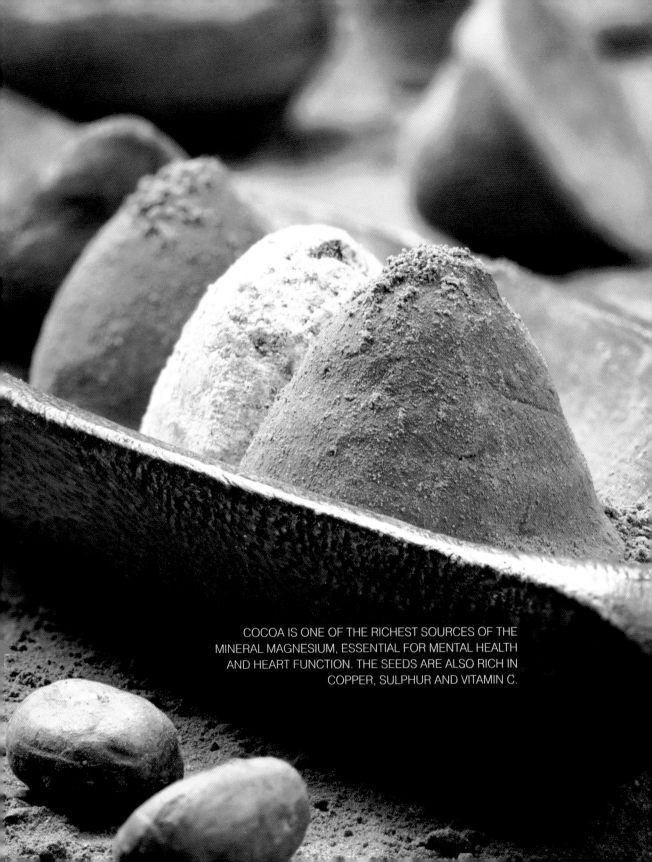

COCOA IS ONE OF THE RICHEST SOURCES OF THE
MINERAL MAGNESIUM, ESSENTIAL FOR MENTAL HEALTH
AND HEART FUNCTION. THE SEEDS ARE ALSO RICH IN
COPPER, SULPHUR AND VITAMIN C.

RED WINE

Red Wine made a big entry into the 'it's good for you' books about 10 years ago when it was discovered it had good levels of the antioxidant resveratrol. Resveratrol is a natural chemical compound found in grapes, more specifically the skin of red grapes and grape seeds. This is why they say red wine is better for you than white. Resveratrol has been promoted as a treatment for many conditions—including ageing itself. A glass of red wine not only gives you a feeling of wellbeing, studies also reveal it can lower bad (LDL) cholesterol by as much as 46 per cent, while increasing good (HDL) cholesterol by up to 24 per cent. Just don't go overboard!

Now, before you go and crack open a Cabernet Sauvignon, remember wine has a very high sugar content and contains a fair amount of alcohol—the amount of both is dependent on the fermentation process. Also, your body cannot store alcohol, so it stays circulating in the blood and becomes the priority fuel over everything else, even the stored glucose (glycogen) in your muscles. For this reason, going for a run after drinking a lot of alcohol is a great way to burn off the alcohol and help avoid or reduce symptoms of a hang-over. Ironically, it is probably the last thing you feel like doing!

Most wine has preservatives added to it as well, not to mention the chemicals used in the grape growing process, so while you are on the Get Clean program it is ideal not to succumb to a glass of wine or other alcoholic beverages. If you must, no more than two glasses per WEEK. Think of a glass of wine as a cup of sugar. And we all know how bad sugar is!

THE RED WINE WITH THE MOST BENEFITS

MUSCADINE
Muscadine grapes, native to south-east United States, are rich in the phenolic compounds, ellagic acid and catechins that stimulate antioxidant activity. According to a study conducted by professors at the University of Florida, muscadine wine may contain three to four times more beneficial phenolic compounds than wine made from California grapes.

PINOT NOIR
Resveratrol is an antioxidant enzyme found in the skin of grapes grown in cool climates. Pinot noir contains more resveratrol than any other red wine. Regions that produce the best pinot noirs include the Willamette Valley in Oregon, the Marlborough region of New Zealand and the Burgundy region of France.

CABERNET SAUVIGNON
Cabernet Sauvignon wine has a high content of procyanidins, a group of compounds found in grape seed extract. Procyanidins make other antioxidants, such as vitamin C and vitamin E, more effective. The body absorbs them easily, and they provide antioxidant protection to the brain and the nervous system.

MADIRAN
Madiran red wine, originally grown in southwestern France, is also considered to be one of the healthiest red wines. It is made of tannat grapes and the long fermentation times and extensive maceration processes used to produce Madiran red wine enhance its healthful properties.

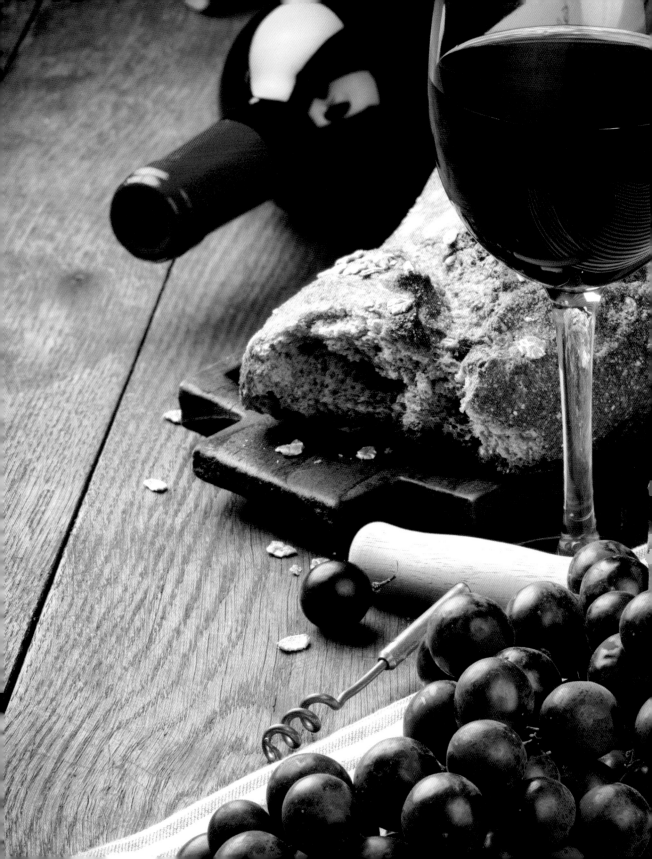

ANTIOXIDANT OVERVIEW

CLASS/COMPONENTS	SOURCE	POTENTIAL BENEFIT
Carotenoids		
Beta-carotene	apricots, butternut squash, cantaloupe, carrots, sweet potatoes, spinach,	Neutralises free radicals and supports cellular antioxidant defenses
Lutein, Zeaxanthin	citrus fruits, collards, corn, eggs, kale, spinach	Contributes to maintenance of healthy vision
Lycopene	tomatoes and tomato products	Contributes to maintenance of prostate health
Flavonoids		
Anthocyanidin	berries, cherries, red grapes	Supports cellular antioxidant defenses; may contribute to maintenance of brain function
Flavanols—Catechin, Epicatechin, Procyanidin	apples, chocolate, cocoa, grapes, tea	Contributes to maintenance of heart health
Flavanones	citrus foods	Neutralise free radicals and supports cellular antioxidant defenses
Flavonols	apples, broccoli, onions, tea	Neutralise free radicals and supports cellular antioxidant defenses
Proanthocyanidin	apples, cinnamon, cocoa, cranberries, grapes, peanuts, strawberries, wine	Contributes to maintenance of urinary tract health and heart health
Isothiocyanates		
Sulforaphane	broccoli, broccoli sprouts, cabbage, cauliflower, kale, horseradish	Enhances detoxification of free radicals and supports cellular antioxidant defences
Phenols		
Caffeic acid, Ferulic acid	apples, citrus fruits, pears, some vegetables	Bolster cellular antioxidant defenses; may contribute to maintenance of healthy vision and heart health
Sulfides/Thiols		
Diallyl sulfide, Allyl methyl trisulfide	garlic, leeks, onions, scallions	Enhance detoxification and contributes to maintenance of heart health and healthy immune function
Dithiolthiones	cruciferous vegetables—broccoli, bok choy, cabbage, collard greens	Contributes to maintenance of healthy immune function

Adapted from International Food Information Council Foundation: Media Guide on Food Safety and Nutrition. 2004-2006. Please note that this is not a representation of all sources or types of antioxidants.

CLASS/COMPONENTS	SOURCE	POTENTIAL BENEFIT
Vitamins		
Vitamin A	dairy products, fish, liver	Protects cells from free radicals
Vitamin C	bell peppers/capsicums, citrus fruits	Protects cells from free radicals
Vitamin E	mixed nuts, oils, sunflower seeds	Protects cells from free radicals, helps with immune function and DNA repair
Selenium	Brazil nuts, meats, plant foods, tuna	Helps prevent cellular damage from free radicals

Antioxidants are of many types and are found in an abundance of foods. This table only highlights a few of them. The main thing you need to know is that fruit and vegetables are loaded with them and while you are on the Get Clean Get Lean program you will be eating a lot of these foods, especially vegetables. I'll even have you addicted to green juices and smoothies—I know, it doesn't sound appetising now, but you are about to be wooed.

Also, you can see the main role of antioxidants is to mop up the free radicals in our blood. This, in simplistic terms, means they clean things up and reduce your toxic load. Toxins in your body cause inflammation, ageing and, at worst, cancer. So, eat, drink and bathe in these foods.

I cannot stress enough how important it is that these foods make up at least 50 per cent of your diet. You are not meant to go hungry while doing the cleanse. If you are, eat these antioxidant-rich foods, or have a veggie-based smoothie and add some nuts and seeds to help satisfy your hunger. This is not a starvation diet, rather a program designed to reduce your toxins, your toxic exposure, nurture your vital organs and leave you feeling absolutely fantastic.

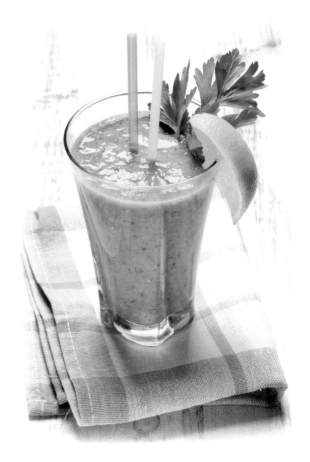

SUPERFOODS

Not all food is created equal and some food should come wearing a cape since their power is so great. These foods are commonly known as superfoods. As their name implies, they are super dense with nutrients and super healthy for you. They are loaded with antioxidants, are low GI, low HI, and contain the good fats. In Europe, they go by the term functional food, a concept originally conceived in Japan, rather than superfood. Superfood or 'functional foods' go over and beyond when it comes to nourishing the body. They also play a role in improving your health and preventing or reducing the risk of disease.

Depending on who you follow, will depend on what foods are on the Top 10 Super or Functional Food list. Most lists contain food choices whose nutritional value has been long recognised. For example, these would be berries, nuts and seeds in general, dark green vegetables (such as kale, collard greens, Swiss chard, Brussels sprouts and broccoli), citrus fruits, fatty fish such as salmon, mackerel and sardines, vegetables with bright, dark or intense colours (such as beets and their greens, and sweet potatoes), certain wild mushrooms, many legumes (peanuts, lentils, beans, raw cocoa), and whole grains as a group.

However, more recently foods like acai, camu camu and goji berries, chia and hemp seeds, bee pollen, figs and maca have been present on more and more lists. I love the work of David Wolfe, who has been a pioneer in this area, particularly getting obscure foods out of the closet and onto dinner plates and into juices and smoothies. I barely make a smoothie or a batch of muffins without adding chia seeds. Here's a list of superfoods my friend and awesome healthy chef, Teresa Cutter (thehealthychef.com) has created. Eat and enjoy them in abundance as they should be a large part of your daily food intake (water too)!

AVOCADO

Avocados are high in fat, but much of this fat is the good monounsaturated type, which resists oxidation and helps neutralise fat in other foods. Research also suggests that eating avocado can improve your cholesterol levels. They are a great source of Vitamin E, C and potassium.

I like to add avocado to many of my salads. Mix chopped avocado with poached organic chicken or jumbo shrimp/king prawns and finish off with chopped cilantro/coriander, scallion/spring onion and a light dressing made from lime juice, fish sauce, honey, garlic and chilli. Avocados also make fantastic, healthy dressings and dips. Blend with a little lime juice, honey, garlic, water, sea salt and cracked pepper for a delicious, healthy dressing for chicken, seafood and leafy salads.

BEANS AND PULSES

Studies indicate that regular consumption of beans and pulses, particularly lentils and soybeans, reduces the risk of cancer. Soybeans are an excellent source of low-fat protein and are included in foods such as miso, soymilk, tofu and tempeh.

Cooked red lentils make great healthy veggie burgers—just make a dhal and add grated carrot, finely chopped celery and fresh herbs, then stiffen the mix with some wheat germ (or ground almonds, if you're intolerant to wheat or gluten). Dip in lightly beaten egg white and coat with more ground almonds. Spray lightly with olive oil and bake in a hot oven, or gently pan fry, until golden.

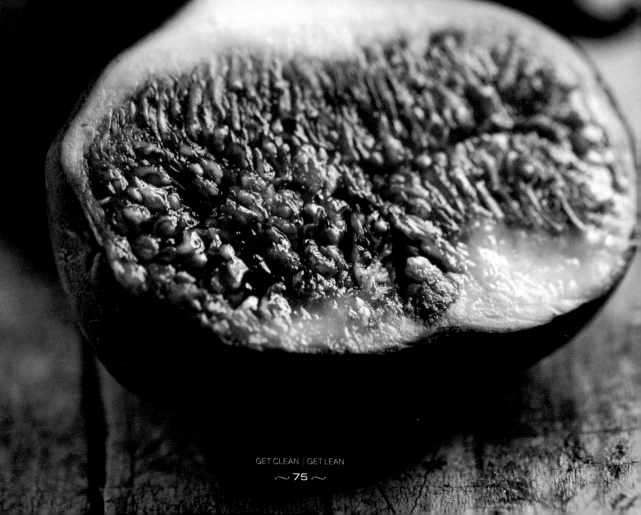

Figs are one of the highest plant sources of calcium and fibre, and contain potassium, magnesium, Vitamin B6 and antioxidants. They are rich in iron, copper and contain traces of zinc, with a mineral content much higher than most other fresh foods. Only cheese and a few nuts have a higher calcium content. They can be included in sweet or savoury dishes, or enjoyed simply on their own. One raw fig has about 40 calories, no cholesterol and no fat. Japanese researchers have discovered that figs contain a natural chemical called benzaldehyde that has been so effective in fighting cancer that it has been added to several medications in Europe and Japan.

BROCCOLI

Broccoli provides an awesome array of antioxidants, including Vitamin C and beta-carotene, which help protect against cancer and other diseases. It is also rich in folate and high in fibre, providing maximum protection from disease when eaten raw or lightly cooked.

I like to make a delicious raw broccoli salad by finely chopping broccoli and adding chopped cilantro/coriander, scallion/spring onion, raw seeds and nuts, then finishing off with a dressing made from tahini, lime juice, honey and miso.

BERRIES

Acai berries, blueberries, raspberries, blackberries, cranberries—all contain a whopping amount of antioxidants. Both blueberries and cranberries also help ward off urinary tract infections.

Berries are delicious in all sorts of salads and desserts, and add moisture and little pockets of flavour to any healthy cake or muffin mix. For a quick breakfast, lightly spread sugar-free blueberry jam and low-fat ricotta on toasted rye bread, then top with sliced banana, blueberries and raw almonds. Yum!

CABBAGE

Cabbage contains great anti-cancer and antioxidant compounds. One study found that those who ate cabbage once a week, compared with once a month, had only 66 per cent of the risk of colon cancer. Eaten raw or lightly cooked, it is an excellent source of Vitamin C and dietary fibre.

For a light and healthy low-carb lunch or dinner, make a tasty, low-fat coleslaw with coconut and lime dressing and serve with grilled or poached organic chicken. Stir-fry lightly in a little stock, finish off with a dash of oyster sauce and top with shredded omelette.

Acai has one of the highest antioxidant contents in the world, neutralises free radicals, contains high levels of essential fatty acids, helps regenerate stem cells, has a very low GI, and fights cancer. Unfortunately, it is hard to get fresh and is generally put in drinks and then loaded up with sugar. If you are buying a pre-mixed acai product, read the label and ask about the added sugar—usually there's a lot!

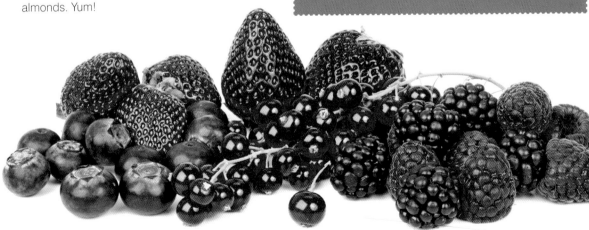

CARROTS

High in Vitamins A and C, and packed with beta-carotene, carrots are legendary in fighting off ageing diseases. People with low levels of beta-carotene in their blood are more prone to heart attack, stroke and various cancers. Studies have also shown that eating a couple of carrots a day can lower blood cholesterol by 10 per cent.

Carrots are easy to incorporate into recipes. Just add chopped carrots to a pot of stock for a simple and delicious creamy carrot soup. Or lightly steam and toss with honey and oven-roasted sesame seeds. For a delicious, healthy salad, mix grated carrot with tahini, miso and mirin, then fold in a few raw seeds and nuts.

CITRUS FRUIT

The orange is 'the complete package' when it comes to natural anti-cancer inhibitors. An excellent source of Vitamin C, which helps make the collagen that is essential for healthy skin, oranges also help maintain the body's defence against bacterial infections. Another great citrus fruit is grapefruit, which has a unique type of fibre that can dramatically reduce cholesterol, protecting against atherosclerosis.

Citrus fruit is fantastic in all sorts of salads. Try oranges and pink grapefruit with a drizzle of raw honey and a sprinkle of pistachio nuts. Or serve the segments with crisp salad leaves, crunchy walnuts and sliced fresh dates.

FISH

Omega-3 fatty acid is the first thing that comes to mind when I think of fish. The human body cannot manufacture this essential fatty acid on its own, so we need to consume small amounts in our diet. Research suggests that this polyunsaturated fat may help prevent against cardiovascular disease, high cholesterol and heart attack. Omega-3s also inhibit adult-onset diabetes, some skin diseases and rheumatoid arthritis. Good sources of omega-3 are found in fish like salmon, swordfish, anchovy, herring, mackerel, sardines and tuna.

Lightly cook a piece of tuna, flake it through a fragrant lettuce salad comprising shredded iceberg, grated carrot and bean sprouts. Finish off with a light dressing made with lime juice, fish sauce, sweet chilli sauce and raw honey. Topped onto whole grain toast, sardines make a delicious, quick and easy, high protein breakfast or snack. Or lightly poach salmon in a little chicken stock and serve on steamed green beans with a squeeze of lemon and a sprinkling of fresh garden herbs.

GINGER, TURMERIC AND BLACK PEPPER

Ginger is great for circulation and nausea, turmeric acts as an anti-inflammatory and antioxidant for the liver, while black pepper helps stabilise blood sugar. These all pack a powerful punch of health benefits and flavour to your cooking, without the use of too much fat.

GRAPES

Red and black grapes contain 20 known antioxidants that work together to fend off free radicals. The antioxidants are in the skin, so the more colourful the skin, the more antioxidants.

If you're craving lollies and chocolate, these are a fantastic alternative sugar fix. Add to fruit salads or freeze and eat frozen for delicious home-made mini icy treats.

GREEN TEA

Rich in antioxidants, studies show that people who consume 1–2 cups of green tea per day have a lower risk of certain cancers.

ONION AND GARLIC

They might give you bad breath, but they also help prevent cancer, thin your blood by discouraging clots and raise the good type (HDL) of cholesterol. They also have antibacterial and anti-inflammatory qualities, helping keep colds and flu at bay. Next time you have a bad case of the flu, try mashing a whole bulb of raw garlic and eating it spread on a piece of wholegrain bread (but preferably not when you're going to be in contact with too many people!). These beauties are fantastic thrown into salad, soup, hearty low-fat casseroles and stir-fries.

SEAWEED

When talking vegetables, we mustn't forget the important benefits of sea vegetables. The most common varieties are kombu, used in soups and stews, wakame, which is normally found in miso soup, and nori, which is the kind used for wrapping sushi rolls. They are all rich in essential minerals and studies have found they are effective in helping prevent a variety of cancers. Try to add seaweed to your stocks, salads, soups, vegetable dishes and casseroles. They are great as a crispy snack too.

SPINACH AND KALE

Green, leafy vegetables top the list of foods most eaten by people who don't get cancer. They are a super source of antioxidants and are high in folate.

Serve simply with a drizzle of lemon and flaxseed oil with poached fish. Or toss with Thai aromatics like lemongrass, chilli, lime juice and honey and serve with organic chicken sprinkled with oven-roasted cashew nuts. Or blanch some spinach until wilted, then chop and add to veggie pies, creamy low-fat risottos or just drizzle with a little soy sauce and mirin to eat as a warm salad.

TOMATOES

Tomatoes are the richest source of lycopene, which forms the red pigment in the flesh. New research suggests that lycopene may help preserve mental and physical functioning among the elderly and reduce the risk of prostate, pancreatic and cervical cancer.

Tomatoes make delicious, fat-free pasta sauces. Or for a yummy, low-carb breakfast, grill and serve with scrambled egg whites and mushrooms. Lightly drizzle roasted tomatoes with good quality balsamic and serve with rocket leaves, low-fat feta and grilled fish. Very delicious and very healthy!

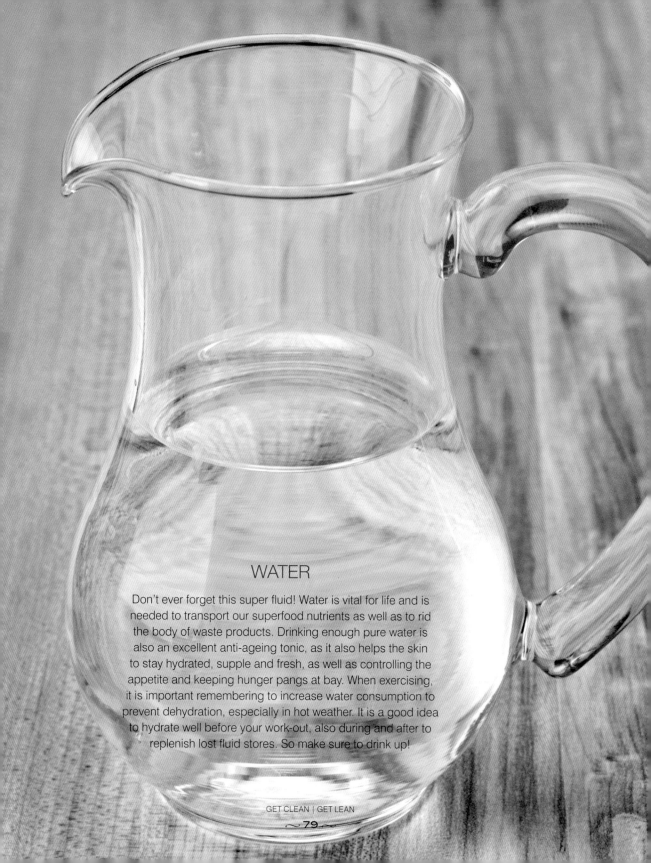

WATER

Don't ever forget this super fluid! Water is vital for life and is needed to transport our superfood nutrients as well as to rid the body of waste products. Drinking enough pure water is also an excellent anti-ageing tonic, as it also helps the skin to stay hydrated, supple and fresh, as well as controlling the appetite and keeping hunger pangs at bay. When exercising, it is important remembering to increase water consumption to prevent dehydration, especially in hot weather. It is a good idea to hydrate well before your work-out, also during and after to replenish lost fluid stores. So make sure to drink up!

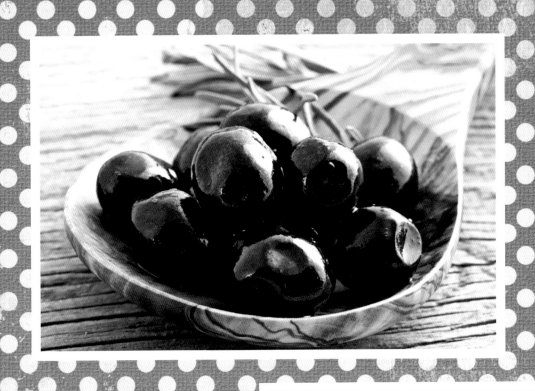

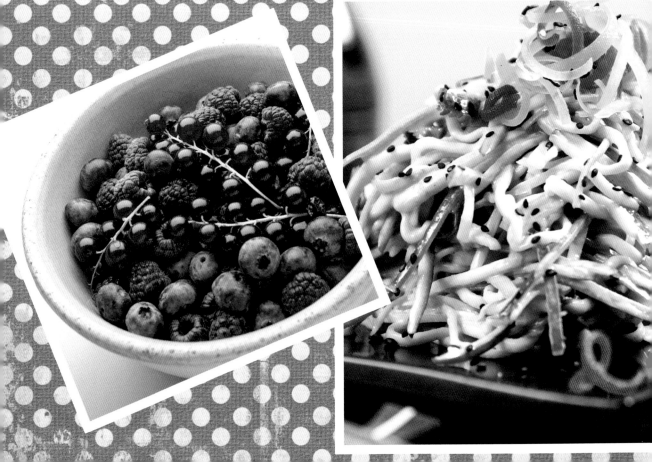

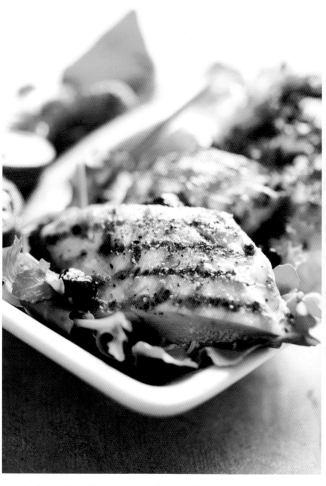

Understanding the benefits and costs of what you put in your body helps you eat healthy. It's a bit like when you are pregnant, all of a sudden you think twice about what you put in your mouth and the health consequences of that. Just remind yourself there is something special growing inside your body that you need to nurture—it's you!

So, if you'e ready, and feel you are armed with the right ammunition, let's do this. Let's get rid of the toxins in your body, let's feed it like it's the most important thing in your world (actually ... it is!) and let's get you healthy for good.

One last thing: there is no point preparing and having all this glorious, vital, colourful, nutritious food in front of you if you are not going to eat it right. SLOW food and mindful eating go hand in hand. Take time out to eat and be conscious of every spoonful you put in your mouth. Chew it, enjoy it and feel what it does to your body.

OK. Now you are ready to Get Ready.

Digestion starts in the mouth. The more you liquidise food in your mouth, the better it will be absorbed in your stomach and intestine. To avoid poor digestion, it is important not to overload your mouth or stomach. In addition, the more thoroughly you chew food, the longer it takes you to eat, so you're more likely to notice when you're full and will therefore eat less. Many people say they no longer hear the hormonal message the body sends to our brain telling us to stop eating. So often we bolt our food before the message reaches our brain, and we have overeaten again. Overeating can lead to poor digestion and obesity.

Just one last thing ... a reminder of how much food you should eat. In 2002, the US National Institutes of Health (NIH) published new nutritional guidelines. We like the NIH's figures in part because they allow for individual tailoring. Specifically, they advised the following ranges:

* Carbohydrate: 45–65 per cent of energy
* Fat: 25–35 per cent of energy
* Protein: 15–35 per cent of energy

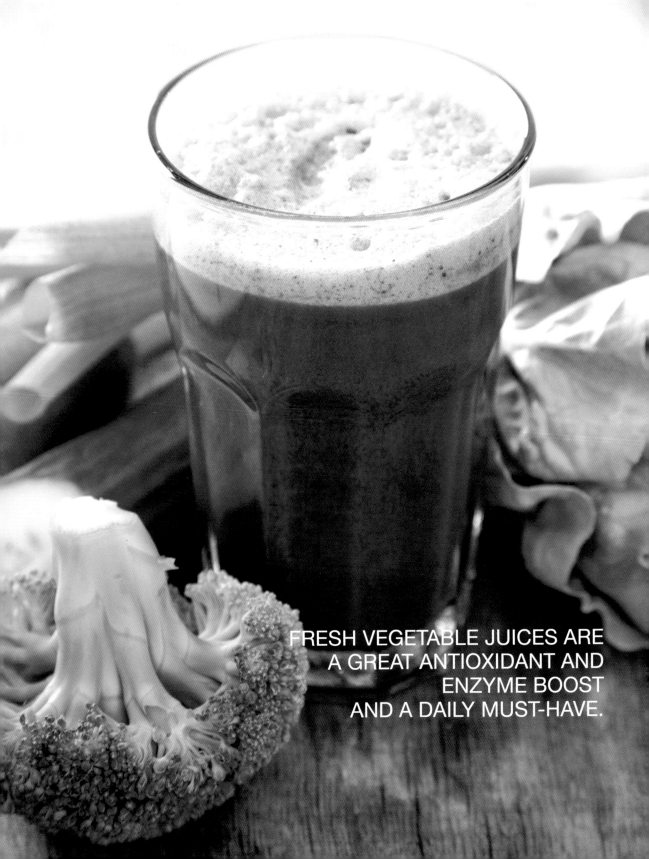

FRESH VEGETABLE JUICES ARE
A GREAT ANTIOXIDANT AND
ENZYME BOOST
AND A DAILY MUST-HAVE.

GET READY

Before you start the four-week Get Clean Get Lean program, and to help you to get the best outcome possible, there are a few things you can do leading up to the start of the program:

* Try to slowly wean yourself off your toxic vices. Cut back (with the view to eliminate) alcohol, coffee, cigarettes, refined carbohydrates (such as white rice, white pasta), sugars, chocolate, lollies, sweets, trans and saturated fats, artificial flavours and sweeteners, and foods loaded with preservatives.
* Minimise the use of chemical-based household cleaners and personal health care products (cleansers, shampoos, deodorants, make-up and toothpastes) and substitute with natural alternatives.
* Try to reduce your stress level, which triggers your body to release stress hormones into your system. While these hormones can provide the adrenaline rush to win a race or meet a deadline, in large amounts they create toxins and slow down detoxification enzymes in the liver. Yoga, meditation and taking time out for you, are great ways to help reduce and manage stress.
* Get rid of any foods or beverages that might tempt you during your cleanse. It's harder to have a chocolate if it's not in the house.
* Drink more water. Your body needs plenty of water to flush out toxins during your cleanse and it will keep you hydrated. Drink at least 2 litres (8 glasses) of filtered water per day.
* To enhance relaxation as you detox, consider buying some essential oils to add to your bathwater or use for massage. Incredibly calming, lavender oil may be especially helpful for those suffering from caffeine-withdrawal-related headaches.

WATER WISE

+ Drink 2–3 litres of purified water every day (more if you have a good sweat).

+ Store your water in glass or stainless steel bottles.

+ Add flavour to your water with fresh sliced lemon, lime, orange, mint or basil leaves.

+ Drink herbal tea instead of coffee or black tea, which have a diuretic effect.

+ Leave a water jug on your desk at work to remind you to drink water.

+ If you're dehydrated, you will feel sluggish. Drnk a few glasses of water and feel your vitallity return.

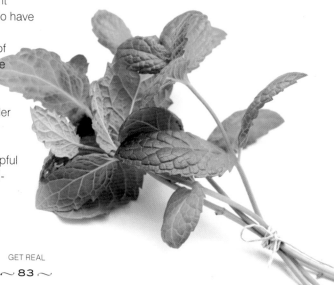

THINGS TO GET RID OF

I know, it goes against every grain in your body to toss out perfectly good food, however if you want to get clean it's time to get ruthless. You are going to give your cupboards or pantry and fridge a detox! You must toss out all tempting and offending items in your cupboard and fridge and make room for all the good foods you need to stock up on. Grab some boxes or grocery bags and start tossing. Keeping secret stashes of unhealthy food 'just in case' is planning for failure; you want to plan for success. Plus I've got some great recipes that will satisfy those sweet cravings, while nourishing you at the same time.

To alleviate any feelings of guilt you may have about throwing out good food, take any unopened, unexpired items to your local homeless shelter or food bank. While this stuff is not the most nourishing food, some people are in situations where something is better than nothing.

STEP ONE

Toss any expired items or open containers into the rubbish or recycling bin. Scan all food in your pantry, fridge and freezer and toss it if it's expired.

Toss: Anything with the word 'hydrogenated' or 'trans fat' in the ingredients list.

Toss: Any food that contains the word 'BHT' or food colouring (e.g. Red 40, Yellow 5) in the ingredients list.

Toss: Any food that contains the word 'enriched' in the ingredients list.

Toss: Any food that contains high-fructose corn syrup in the ingredients list.

Toss: Any food that contains artificial sweeteners (aspartame, saccharine, and acesulfame potassium, Splenda, NutriSweet, Equal).

STEP TWO

Next you will attack your pantry or cupboard where you keep non-perishables.

Toss: All junk food. Doritos, chips, Twisties, Oreos, processed cookies, lollies etc. You know what this stuff is, so even though I haven't listed it, you know what junk food is. Keep pure dark chocolate that is at least 70 per cent cocoa.

Toss: Any peanut butter that isn't organic and/or contains more ingredients than just peanuts on the label (e.g. Kraft and most generic brands)

Toss: All grain products that have the word 'enriched' in the ingredients list. This is probably almost if not all grain products you have (e.g. bread, pasta, crackers, and cereal like Cheerios, Special K, Weet-bix and Cornflakes).

Toss: All white bread, white flour, refined bread-like products (e.g. pitas, crumpets, muffins etc.)

Toss: Crisco, margarine and other unhealthy baking products.

Toss: Agave nectar (Or, you can keep it and use it in very strict moderation.)

Toss: Maple syrup that contains corn syrup. (100% pure maple syrup is OK to keep.)

Toss: Any kind of meal that comes in a can (e.g. soup, spaghetti, baked beans etc).

Toss: Almost all canned fruits and vegetables. Cans that are OK to keep: organic tomato products, organic beans, vegetarian refried beans, organic coconut milk and artichoke hearts packed in water.

AS A GENERAL RULE, IF THERE ARE NUMBERS LISTED IN THE INGREDIENTS PANEL, TOSS!

STEP 3

Next we go to the refrigerator door where the condiments and spreads are kept.

Toss: All store-bought salad dressing.

Toss: Soy sauce, non-organic ketchup (it most likely contains high-fructose corn syrup) and commercial jams and spreads.

Toss: Anything with high-fructose corn syrup, the word 'hydrogenated' on the label, food colouring and/or BHT (or other preservatives).

STEP 4

Use the rules in steps 1–3 to scan your refrigerator for unhealthy items and toss them. If any fresh produce has been there more than 10 days, toss that too. Are you starting to see a lot of clear space?

STEP 5

Move to the freezer and toss the bad stuff.

Toss: Ice cream and other frozen sweets.

Toss: Microwavable meals, TV dinners, anything with preservatives in it.

STEP 6

Double-check your spice cabinet. Spice cabinets can be a graveyard for expired food. Look at your oils, vinegars and spices, and toss anything expired and take a mental note of what you're throwing out. Next time, buy just what you need. Most natural food stores will let you buy spices in bulk or small quantities (e.g. if you don't use cardamom a lot and want it for a recipe, just buy wthat you need instead of an entire bottle.)

Toss: Spices that contain preservatives and/or food colouring.

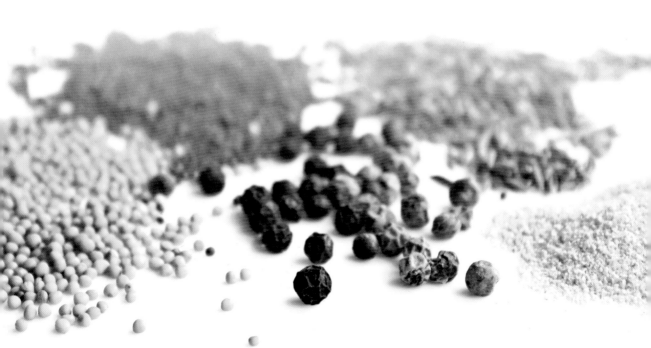

THINGS TO STOCK UP ON

Now that you have given your cupboards, pantry and fridge a good cleanse, it is time to restore them with healthy, clean food. Below is a list of basic things I keep on hand, not necessarily all at once. Purchasing all of these items is not required, just work within your budget and stock up on what you love and know you eat on a regular basis. Remember to pay attention to expiration dates and don't purchase more than you'll use by that date. Fresh is best. That said, I often stock up on frozen berries as they can be hard to get and expensive in winter. Just check on the label that they have been snap frozen and have nothing added.

Beans, grains, canned goods and frozen items are inexpensive and shelf-stable, so feel free to buy a lot to have on hand. Always buy without added sugar and salt, and the organic option if you can. I didn't include fresh produce here as that's something you'll buy fresh every few days as you need it. The main thing is to buy food in its most natural state possible, without added chemicals (mainly flavours and presrvatives). Buy nuts raw and unsalted, oils cold-pressed, and wherever possible, go for the organic options. This will mean less toxic exposure and will make your cleanse more efficeint. Also, always read labels: if they have words you can't pronounce or numbers, pop the item back on the store shelf.

Low GI Grains	Canned Food	Frozen Food	Nuts, Seeds & Pulses	Meat & Eggs
Quinoa	Black beans	Organic edamame (shelled or not, your preference)	Raw almonds	Organic eggs
Whole rolled or steel cut oats	Kidney beans		Raw walnuts	Organic chicken and turkey breast
Long-grain brown rice (not quick cooking)	White beans (a.k.a. cannellini beans)	Organic frozen peas	Raw sunflower seeds (out of shell)	Fresh ocean fish
	Chickpeas	Organic frozen whole corn	Raw pumpkin seeds	Lean beaf and lamb
100% whole grain pasta (not wheat)	Diced tomatoes	Frozen berries (organic if you can)	Organic, ground flax seeds	No cold cuts or deli meats
Quinoa or brown rice pasta	Tomato sauce	Any other frozen fruit that looks good	Chia seeds	
100% sprouted grain bread	Albacore tuna (sustainably caught)		Your favorite nut butter (e.g. almond butter (or 100% natural peanut butter)	
Wholegrain sourdough			Lentils	

Dairy & Milks	Oils	Vinegar & Condiments	Herbs & Spices	Sweeteners
Goat's milk cheese	Preferably organic and cold-pressed:	Raw apple cider vinegar (keep in the refrigerator)	Freshly ground black pepper	100% real stevia (I prefer the liquid Sweet Leaf brand)
Unsweetened Greek yogurt. (pay attention to expiration dates)	Organic extra virgin olive oil	Aged balsamic vinegar	Himalayan pink salt	Grade B maple syrup
Organic unsalted butter	Organic raw, virgin coconut oil (a.k.a. coconut butter)	Red wine vinegar	Ground cumin	Raw honey (local to you is best)
Unsweetened almond milk (or nut milk of choice)	Cold-pressed flax seed oil	Dijon mustard	Chilli powder	Your favorite real fruit jam (low sugar, 100% natural)
Coconut water	Sesame oil	Tamari (tamari is a gluten-free soy sauce)	Cinnamon	Barley malt
Coconut milk	Macadamia nut oil (expensive but worth it—great butter substitute)	Real vegetable stock	Garlic salt	Brown rice syrup
	Avocado oil	Home-made pesto	Crushed red pepper flakes	No artificial sweeteners, EVER!
		Tahini	Dried basil and oregano	
		Hummus	Dried bay leaves	
			Pure vanilla extract (or whole beans)	
			Turmeric (expensive, buy in small qualities)	

WIPE EVERY DOWN AND MAKE ROOM FOR THE GOOD STUFF — CLEAN FOOD!

WHY BUY ORGANIC?

This is a good question, with many good answers. When I asked myself this question, the answer came easily. For me, buying organic anything is about health. I have worked in the health industry for over 25 years in the areas of fitness and nutrition and I'm always looking to find ways for our bodies to operate at their optimum level. My main concern is that pesticides, herbicides, fertilisers and antibiotic residues have a habit of creeping into our food— and what doesn't creep in during cultivation tends to get added during further processing. On any given day, the average person consumes well over 30 harmful chemicals. And this is not healthy!

AN OUNCE OF PREVENTION IS WORTH A POUND OF CURE!

Originally, all foods were 'organic'. They were grown and prepared without pesticides, herbicides, chemical fertilisers or irradiation. Food was unrefined, whole, or minimally processed. Since World War II and the advent of chemical farming and food processing, the soils and foods of much of the world have been depleted of many important minerals and nutrients.

Our food these days is not only deficient in nutrients, but also full of pollutants and farming chemicals. The modern process of denaturing foods via heavy refining and chemical treatment deeply affects the life force of our food supply, making it difficult to foster equilibrium and health. Pesticides have been shown to create extra work for the immune system, causing cancer and disease in the liver, kidneys and blood.

Pesticides accumulate in the organs, resulting in a weakened immune system, allowing carcinogens and pathogens to filter into the body.[1] Organic certification is the public's assurance that products have been grown and handled according to strict natural procedures.

A lot of people argue that organic food is more expensive, and I appreciate that as an argument when you have a family to feed. However, I find it hard to put a price on your health! My tip is to buy organic over conventional when buying any of the foods listed in the Dirty Dozen list as these are the most toxic. Also, animal products are worth paying a little more for the organic option. The hormones in chicken meat and cow's milk are meant for their body, not your's! And of course, there's the taste factor. Organic food tastes better. Ask any foodie.

In a unique study conducted over 20 years by Sydney's Royal Prince Alfred Hospital Allergy Clinic and involving more than 20,000 patients, it was found that over 50 food additives are common causes of allergies ranging from skin irritation, headaches and eczema to irritable bowel syndrome, asthma and neurological problems.

There are now over 150 studies linking pesticides with acute and chronic conditions including cancer, neurological damage, reproductive and developmental malfunction, and immune and endocrine disruption.

However, it is scientifically difficult to prove that something causes cancer, since it takes so long to research and there are so many varying factors. For example, it took several decades of research— from the late 1950's to early 1980's—to prove the link between cigarettes and lung cancer, despite the fact that smoking was causing 90% of all lung cancers and 30% of all other cancers. The research continues today.

The best way to avoid food that contains chemicals and additives is to buy food that is organic, or as close to organic as possible.

1. National Resources Defense Council, *Trouble on the Farm: Growing Up with Pesticides in Agricultural Communities*, Chapter 1 http://geti.in/1cSujRE

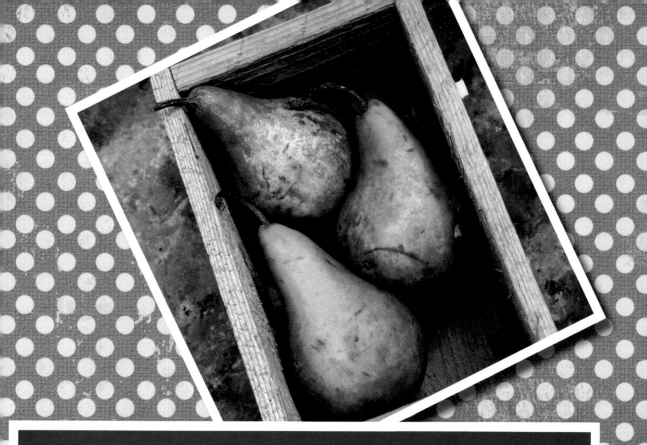

THE DIRTY DOZEN

Buy these organic whenever possible:
* Apples
* Celery
* Sweet bell peppers/capsicums
* Peaches
* Strawberries
* Nectarines—imported
* Grapes
* Spinach
* Lettuce
* Cucumbers
* Blueberries—domestic
* Potatoes

Plus (also buy these organic)
* Green beans
* Kale/Greens

THE CLEAN 15

Lowest in pesticide residue:
* Onions
* Sweet Corn
* Pineapples
* Avocado
* Cabbage
* Sweet peas
* Asparagus
* Mangoes
* Eggplant
* Kiwi
* Cantaloupe/rockmelon—domestic
* Sweet potatoes
* Grapefruit
* Watermelon
* Mushrooms

www.ewg.org/foodnews/summary.php

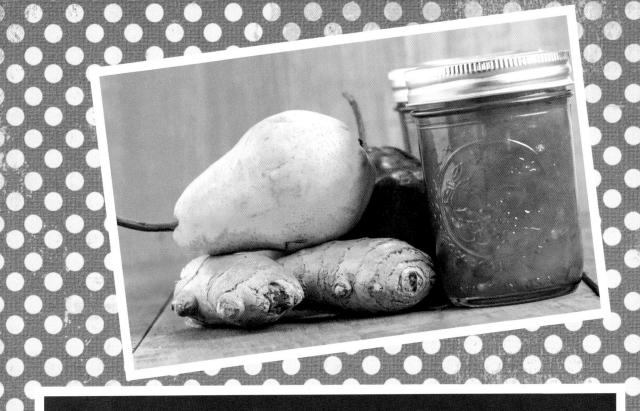

AVOID PLASTIC CONTAINERS

Bisphenol A (BPA) is a chemical used when producing plastic bottles, food containers and the lining of tin cans. BPA can leach out of the plastic and into your food and drink. Once inside your body, BPA can interfere with normal hormonal processes and cause genetic damage, especially in developing foetuses and children. To date, more than 100 studies worldwide have linked BPA with prostate cancer, breast cancer, reproductive disorders and polycystic ovary disease.

WAYS TO REDUCE YOUR RISK

✻   Use containers made of BPA-free plastic, glass or stainless steel.

✻   Check the labels on toys, containers and other plastic items, and look for those that are BPA-free.

✻   Don't put plastics in the microwave as harmful chemicals are much more likely to leach at high temperatures.

✻   Avoid drinking water from plastic bottles and don't reuse disposable plastic water bottles.

✻   Don't use old plastic water bottles as the longer you use the same bottle, the more likely it is that it will start to break down and release toxins.

HOW TO READ FOOD LABELS

Reading food labels can be a tricky business and a little time consuming. But with a bit of know-how, you'll be able to take just a cursory glance at the label and know when it goes in your basket or back on the shelf. Here are the basics consolidated into 10 quick-reference tips, compliments of Dr Gayl Canfield, Director of Nutrition at the Pritikin Longevity Center in Miami, Florida. These 10 tips are all about helping you shed excess weight, take good care of your heart and live well.

1. NEVER BELIEVE THE CLAIMS ON THE FRONT OF THE BOX

What many think are health claims are actually just marketing pitches and advertisements. And government-approved claims, like 'low-fat' and 'light' often don't tell you the whole story. These products may be high in fat as well as sugar, salt, and/or calories. Light ice-cream, for example, may still pack in 4 to 5 grams of fat per serving. And 'light' and 'regular' varieties of ice-cream may not differ much calorically. If you are going to have it, go for the real version.

Never evaluate a product based on any one item, such as its fat, cholesterol, sugar, carbohydrate, or salt content. Attempting to cash in on the latest diet or nutrition craze, many companies promote their products based on a single item despite other unhealthy aspects. (Remember 'fat-free' foods that were full of sugar and calories?) To be truly healthy, a product must pass several criteria.

2. ALWAYS READ THE NUTRITION FACTS LABEL AND THE INGREDIENT LIST

They contain information that can really help you determine how healthy a food is. Crackers, for example, may advertise on the front of the box that they're 'trans fat free', but in the ingredient list you may find fats, like palm oil and coconut oil, that are just as artery-clogging as the trans fats they replaced. And avoid them if there are a bunch of numbers in the list.

3. CHECK THE SERVING SIZE

Though the government standardised most serving sizes years ago, many products still post unrealistically small sizes. A serving of oil spray, for instance, is .25 grams. That's far less than most people could, or would, spray on a pan with even just one squirt.

4. CHECK THE NUMBER OF SERVINGS PER PACKAGE

Decades ago, many products were in fact single servings. A bottle of drink was one serving. One small candy bar was one serving. Today, many products are 'supersized' and contain multiple servings. A 21 fl oz/600 mL bottle of soft drink contains 2.5 servings, at 110 calories each. Now, in the real world, who's going to drink just one serving of that bottle? Is it any surprise that many of us are super-sized ourselves?

5. CHECK THE CALORIES PER SERVING

All too many people think the '110 calories' posted on that 600 mL bottle of soft drink means they're drinking 110 calories. Hardly. You've got to multiply the 110 calories by the total number of servings, 2.5, to realise that you're actually downing a whopping 275 calories.

Don't get too comfortable with '0's either. Because some manufacturers use ridiculously small serving sizes (remember that .25g of cooking spray?) and because the FDA states that manufacturers can 'round down' to zero, some products advertised as calorie-free or fat-free are not. If you eat multiple servings—if, say, you coat an entire skillet with oil spray—you may be tallying up quite a few calories.

6. CHECK THE CALORIES FROM FAT

It's on the Nutrition Facts label. Unfortunately, it doesn't tell you the 'per cent of calories from fat', which is how all health guidelines direct us to limit fat. You've got to do a little math. Divide the number of calories from fat by the total calories. (If the serving is 150 calories, 50 of which are fat, your product is 33 per cent calories from fat.)

If division trips you up, go by grams. Use this easy rule. If a product has 2 grams of fat per 100 calories, the fat, per serving, is 20 per cent of total calories. You don't have to be a mathematician to realise that 4 grams of fat per 100 calories is higher than the rcommended 30 per cent of calories from fat.

Don't be fooled by claims like '99 per cent fat-free' or '2 per cent fat' milk. They're based on percent of weight, not percent of calories. So that can of 99 per cent fat-free soup may actually have 77 per cent of its calories from fat, or more. And 2 per cent fat milk actually has about 34 per cent of total calories from fat; 1 per cent milk has about 23 per cent calories from fat.

7. CHECK THE SODIUM

The best way to see the sodium content is to look at the number of milligrams of sodium the serving contains. A great rule of thumb: Limit the sodium in milligrams to no more than the number of calories in each serving. Your daily goal: less than 1,500 mg of sodium. That's been the daily recommendation for sodium on the Pritikin Program for nearly 40 years, and it is now the recommendation of many leading health authorities, including the American Heart Association and the Centers for Disease Control and Prevention. The Australian National Health and Research Council (NHRC) recommend between 930–2,300 mg of sodium per day. I would advise sticking to the lower end of this RDI.

8. CHECK THE TYPES OF FAT

Make sure there are no saturated fats, partially hydrogenated fats or tropical oils in the ingredient list, including lard, butter, palm oils, shortening, margarine, chocolate, and whole and part-skim dairy products. They're all damaging to your arteries and heart.

Polyunsaturated fats (like safflower, soybean and sesame) and monounsaturated fats (such as olive and canola) are less harmful and would be acceptable, but make sure the per cent calories from fat are still in line—20 per cent calories from fat or less—or your waistline may start getting out of line. All oils, even 'good' oils, are dense with calories.

Watch out for sugars and other caloric sweeteners that don't say 'sugar' but in fact are, such as corn syrup, rice and maple syrup, molasses, honey, malted barley, barley malt, or any term that ends in 'ol', such as sorbitol or maltitol, or 'ose' such as dextrose or fructose.

Try to limit (avoid) all these added, refined, concentrated sugars to no more than 5 per cent of total calories (essentially, no more than 2 tablespoons daily). Don't be concerned about naturally occurring sugars in fruit and some non-fat dairy products. However, on the Nutrition Facts label, added sugars and naturally occurring sugars are all lumped together as 'sugar'.

Your best bet: look at the ingredient list. Try to avoid foods with added, refined caloric sweeteners in the first three to five ingredients. Because ingredients are listed in descending order of weight, the lower down the label you find added sugars, the better.

laboratories evaluated 30 low-carb nutrition bars and found that 60 per cent were inaccurately labelled. Most had more carbs, sugars and salt than their labels claimed.

During your first few trips to the market, give yourself extra time to evaluate products. You'll soon speed up! Once you've found products that you enjoy and that meet these healthy guidelines, shopping becomes quick and easy. Your health is worth it!!

If you are curious about the Australian RDI on all food visit www.nhmrc.gov.au/guidelines/publications/n6.

10. MAKE SURE THAT GRAINS ARE WHOLE GRAIN, SUCH AS WHOLE-WHEAT FLOUR

Many bread and pasta products claim to be whole wheat, but the first ingredient in the ingredient list is often wheat flour, which sounds healthy, but it's really refined flour. Further down the list will be whole-wheat flour or bran. Scout out products that contain only whole grains. And look for at least 3 grams of fibre per serving, which often ensures the product is mostly, if not all, whole grain.

If the product sounds too good to be true, it may be. Thousands of new products come out every year, many trying to cash in on the latest diet craze. Many may not be carefully regulated (if at all). Recently the Florida FDA evaluated 67 diet products and found all 67 were inaccurately labelled; they contained more sugar, for example, than their labels stated. And recently, consumer

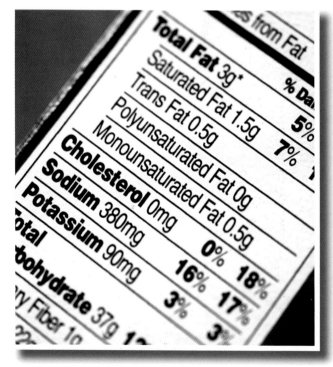

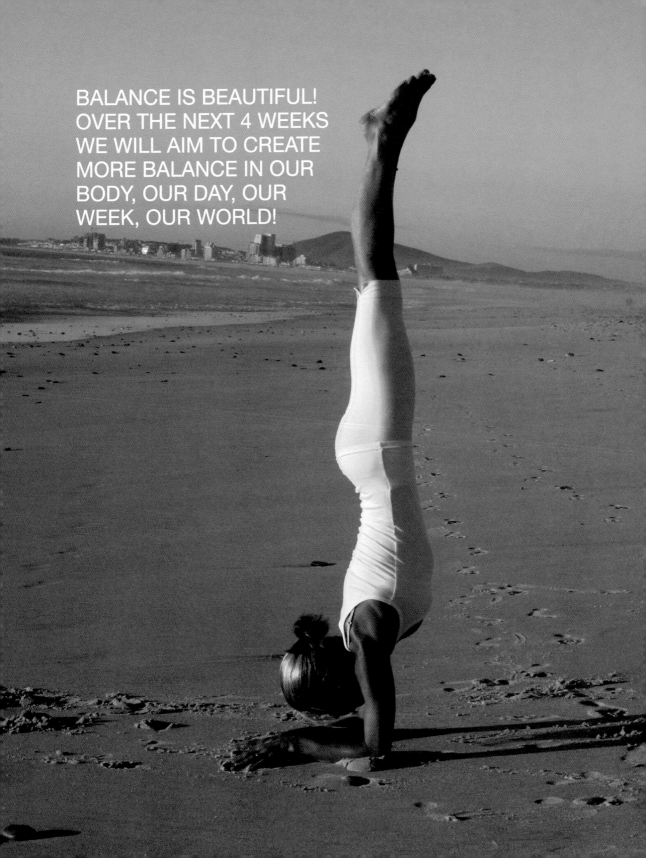

BALANCE IS BEAUTIFUL!
OVER THE NEXT 4 WEEKS
WE WILL AIM TO CREATE
MORE BALANCE IN OUR
BODY, OUR DAY, OUR
WEEK, OUR WORLD!

GET SET

Now is the time for you to change your mind-set about how you feed your body. Treat it like a temple. It is the only body you have ... it will repay you in ways you didn't think were possible. In the words of a very wise man *'Let food be your medicine and medicine be your food. Nature heals: the physician is only nature's assistant.'* (Hippocrates)

In an age where choice is overwhelming, and there is a lot of misinformation about what we should and shouldn't eat, let's make it simple and break it down to two choices: choose foods that provide you with the best possible support biochemically and energetically for health and wellbeing. And choose foods that are irresistibly delicious and colourful.

You've read about nutrition, you've detoxed your cupboards and stocked up on clean food, here are a few last-minute tips before you GO!

Aim to eat at least 50 per cent of your foods in their natural state. When you are under stress, increase this to 75 per cent. From sashimi to strawberries, clean, wholesome foods eaten raw have remarkable health-enhancing and anti-ageing properties. This is why most of the best and most famous spas and health retreats around the world serve raw food for healing and rejuvenation. Uncooked fruit and vegetables improve micro-circulation, cellular functioning and DNA expression. Eating a high percentage of raw food improves your energy and stamina, supplies a high level of bio-photon order to the living matrix, slows ageing and provides you with great antioxidant support.

A QUICK OVER-VIEW OF THE FOUR-WEEK GET CLEAN GET LEAN PROGRAM:

1 Reduce your toxic exposure through a clean diet and lifestyle.

2 Rest and recover your major organs.

3 Remove bad bacteria and toxins from your digestive system.

4 Stimulate the liver to drive toxins from the body.

5 Promote elimination through the intestines, kidneys and skin.

6 Improve circulation of the blood.

7 Refuel your body with healthy, fresh, nutritious, SLOW food.

8 Have you feeling tip-top and restore good health.

10 TIPS FOR CLEAN EATING

1 Try to stay away from grain-based carbs for four weeks. These include flour, breakfast cereals, pasta, breads and all forms of sugar. If this is too hard, add small amounts of whole grains such as brown rice, oats, bread made from rye, oats or spelt, quinoa, amaranth, millet, and buckwheat.

2 Eat an abundance of fresh (preferrably organic) fruit and vegetables every day. Non-starchy vegetables will be your main supply of carbohydrates for the next four weeks. Add small amounts of above if you are feeling tired.

3 Eat at least one big, colourful salad every day. Make it as colourful as you can get and add fresh herbs to give it zing. Sprinkle a good quality protein over the top (nuts, seeds, lean chicken, fish, egg or tofu) and voila!

4 Cut out soft drinks, packaged fruit juces, cordials and alcohol. If you must have the occassional glass of wine, keep it to *no more* than two glasses of quality wine and only indulge once a week. If you can sustain this for four weeks it's worth it.

5 Use cold-pressed extra-virgin olive oil, walnut oil, hazelnut oil and flaxseed oil on your salads. For cooking use butter (yes, that natural stuff that gets a hard wrap), coconut oil or olive oil (these don't convert to trans fats when heated like many vegetable oils).

6 For your protein sources choose raw, unsalted nuts, seeds, free-range eggs and non-GMO soy products. For the non-vegos choose oily fish (no more than three times each week), free-range chicken and turkey and lean cuts of meat.

7 Stay as far away as you can from margarine (even those with added plant sterols that reduce cholesterol). Also avoid processed and highly hydrogenated vegetable oils and any sauces or dressings that contain them. Make your own salad dressings with natural ingredients, fresh herbs, cold pressed oil (above) and a good balsamic vinegar. Remember low HI, and that's for all of your food choices.

8 Eliminate all sugars, including malt extract, corn syrup, and especially those artificial ones (which should be banned along with all those 'diet' drinks that contain them)! If you need a sweetener use manuka honey, grade A maple syrup or stevia (a very sweet herb grown in South America).

9 Drink two litres of water every day. If coffee is a must-have, restrict yourself to one cup a day and drink it unsweetened and black. Same goes for tea. If you do have a black tea or coffee, drink two extra glasses of water to compensate for the diuretic effect these have.

10 If you do succumb to temptation, DO NOT beat yourself up and shower yourself in guilt. Put it behind you and get back on track. Don't use it as an excuse to throw in the towel. Even applying six of these tips is better than nothing. Get back to the why you are doing this, and get on with the doing.

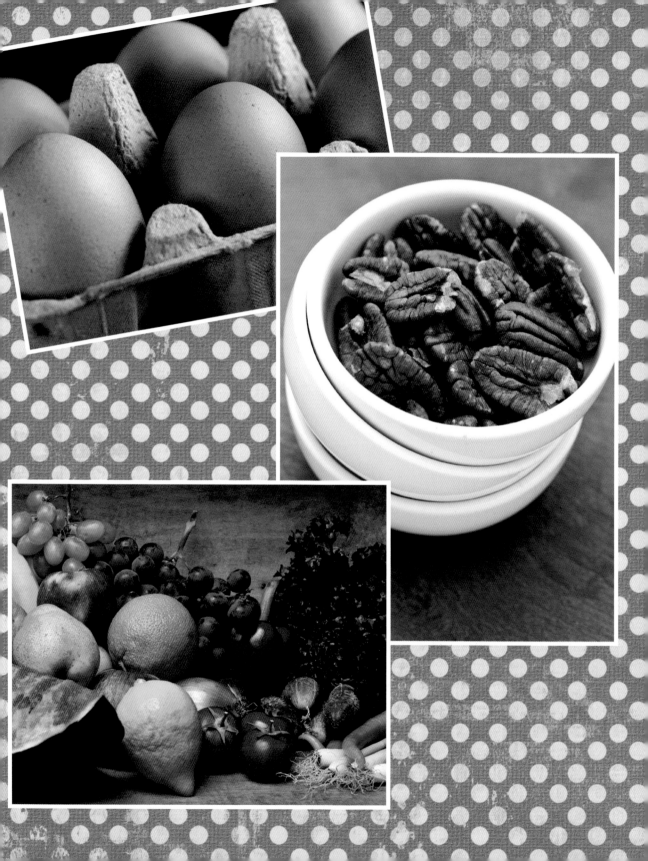

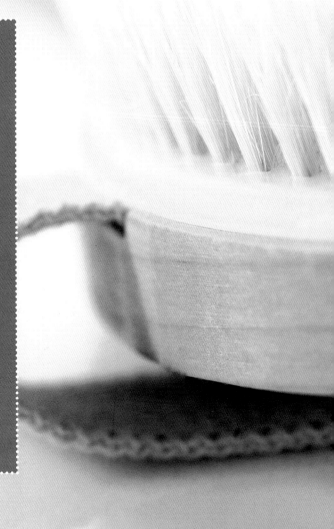

Your skin is the largest organ of your body and should receive a regular detox. Dry brush your skin every day. Start at the extremities and work your way towards your heart. This not only gets rid of dead skin cells, it stimulates blood flow, and helps get rid of cellulite. Also drink plenty of purified water, have a good sweat at least once a day and eat foods that feed your skin such as carrots, avocado, mango, sesame and pumpkin seeds and pears. Simple measures that go a long way in helping you achieve an inner and outer glow!

Try mixing sea salt and avocado oil for a home-made exfoliant. Rub it all over your body (be careful on your face and near your eyes) and wash off in the shower. Your skin will feel silky smooth and supple. Add some essential oils to the mix if you want to smell nice too!

TEN TIPS TO HELP YOUR BODY CLEAN

There are lots of things you can do to help your body clean out the toxins. These practices should become part of your lifestyle to help your body detoxify on an on-going basis.

1 Start each day with a shot of apple cider vinegar (ACV). Mostly I put two tablespoons of vinegar in a mug of hot water and drink it like a tea, but when I'm on the run, a quick shot is the way to go. It stimulates digestive enzymes. Lemon juice in warm water has a similar effect, and a great alternative if the vinegar is too sour for you.

2 Eat plenty of fibre, including brown rice and organically-grown fresh fruits and vegetables. Beets, radishes, artichokes, cabbage, broccoli, spirulina, chlorella, and seaweed are excellent detoxifying foods.

3 Cleanse and protect the liver by taking herbs such as dandelion root, burdock and milk thistle, and drinking green or dandelion tea.

4 Take Vitamin C, which helps the body produce glutathione, a liver compound that drives away toxins.

5 Drink at least two litres of filtered water each day. I know I have stated this before but it is vitally important to good health. With so many people not drinking enough water I feel the message isn't getting through.

6 Breathe deeply to allow oxygen to circulate more completely through your system. This is great for assisting with cleaning your blood. Yoga, meditation and other practices that focus on breathing not only clear the body, but the mind too. Absolute gold if you suffer from stress.

7 Cut yourself some slack. Don't always focus on the negative. Positive affirmations and thoughts (and a big smile) can have a profound affect on your health. More and more research is proving that your mind and body work as one.

8 Treat yourself to a regular massage. This not only stimulates your lymphatic system, but is a great way to reduce tension in your muscles. And I shouldn't call this a treat, it should be a habit!

9 Dry-brush your skin every day before you jump in the shower. This removes dead skin cells so toxins can be removed through the skin more efficiently. It's also very stimulating and great for reducing cellulite.

10 Enjoy daily exercise. A good sweat allows your body to eliminate wastes through perspiration, as well as many other benefits to your mind, body and soul. It's also great for ensuring a good night's sleep.

ONE OF MY LITTLE 'NOT SO DIRTY' SECRETS

My Grandma lived to the ripe old age of 99.9, and for 99 of those years she was in good health. One thing she swore by, and attributed her good health to, was starting each day with a shot of Apple Cider Vinegar (ACV). I have been doing this since I was 13 and it has become a morning ritual I enjoy. Mostly I put 1–2 tablespoons of the vinegar in a mug of hot water and drink it like a tea, but when I'm on the run, a quick shot is the way to go.

They encourage this practise at Gwinganna Lifestyle Retreat to stimulate your digestive enzymes. The shot of vinegar is usually followed by fruit, as many fruits contain digestive enzymes too. This is then followed by breakfast.

Lemon juice in water has a similar effect, and a great alternative if the vinegar is a bit too sour for you. Just thinking about the ACV has my salivary glands working!

HEALTH BENEFITS OF ACV

The Father of Medicine, Hippocrates, used ACV around 400 BC for its health giving qualities. It is said that he had only two remedies: honey and apple cider vinegar.

Apple cider vinegar is made from fresh ripe apples that are fermented and undergo a stringent process to create the final product. The vinegar contains a host of vitamins, beta-carotene, pectin and vital minerals such as potassium, sodium, magnesium, calcium, phosphorous, chlorine, sulphur, iron, and fluorine.

Pectin (a fibre) in the vinegar helps reduce bad cholesterol and plays a role in regulating blood pressure. The vinegar also helps extract calcium from the fruits, vegetables and meat it is mixed with, which is beneficial in maintaining strong bones.

Apple cider vinegar is loaded with potassium. The potassium in this vinegar also helps to eliminate toxic waste from the body. The beta-carotene also helps mop up free radicals assisting the detox process.

It is said to maintain firmer skin and give you a youthful appearance. Hey, I'm not one to argue with the science. If they say that's what it can do ... I am going to believe it with every swig I take.

Apple cider vinegar helps break down fat which helps in natural weight reduction. As above!

It also contains malic acid which is very helpful in fighting fungal and bacterial infections. This acid dissolves uric acid deposits that form around joints, helping relieve joint pains. The dissolved uric acid is gradually eliminated from the body.

It is an acquired taste, and once you're through the cleanse and you need to soften the blow, add some honey. Alternatively, start on a lower dose and work your way up to 2 tablespoons. It is worth it and a super way to start your day.

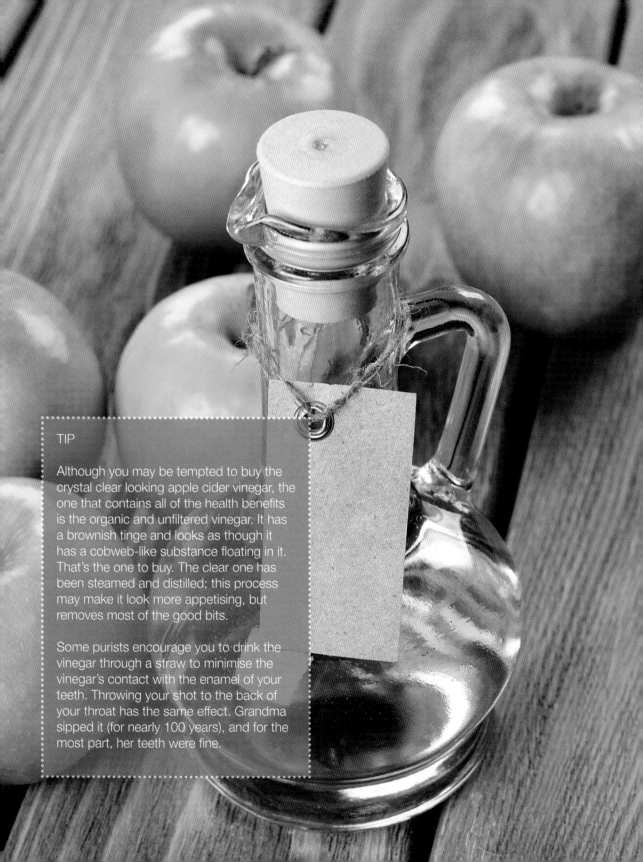

TIP

Although you may be tempted to buy the crystal clear looking apple cider vinegar, the one that contains all of the health benefits is the organic and unfiltered vinegar. It has a brownish tinge and looks as though it has a cobweb-like substance floating in it. That's the one to buy. The clear one has been steamed and distilled; this process may make it look more appetising, but removes most of the good bits.

Some purists encourage you to drink the vinegar through a straw to minimise the vinegar's contact with the enamel of your teeth. Throwing your shot to the back of your throat has the same effect. Grandma sipped it (for nearly 100 years), and for the most part, her teeth were fine.

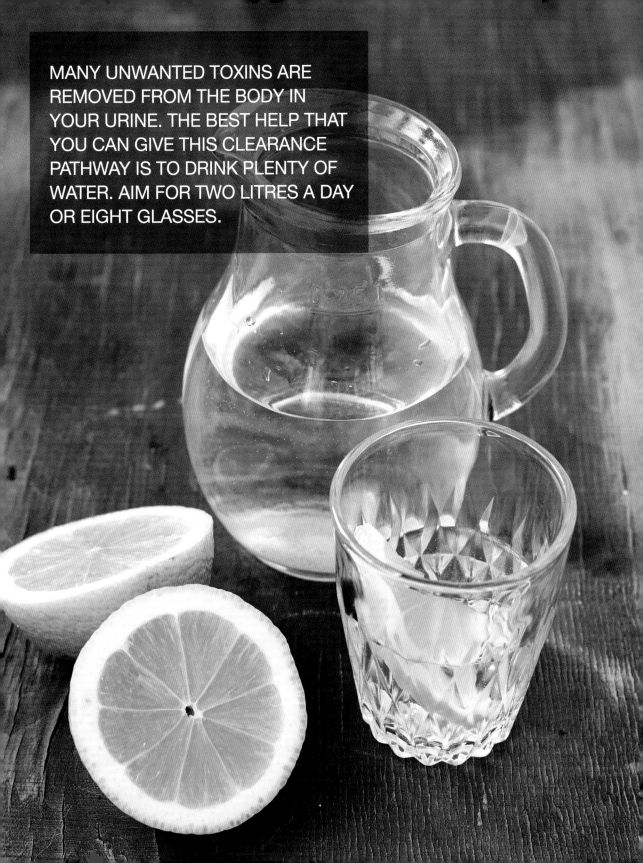

MANY UNWANTED TOXINS ARE REMOVED FROM THE BODY IN YOUR URINE. THE BEST HELP THAT YOU CAN GIVE THIS CLEARANCE PATHWAY IS TO DRINK PLENTY OF WATER. AIM FOR TWO LITRES A DAY OR EIGHT GLASSES.

FOODS TO ENJOY OR AVOID

The following outlines what you should be eating daily from the various food groups and what foods you should avoid. It will arm you with enough information that you can start creating your own meal plans. Personally, I like a program where I can decide what I will eat each day depending on my desire, what's in season, and the time I have to prepare my meals. I know many people prefer the entire diet spelt out for them. If the following information isn't enough for you, go to my blog (krisabbey.com) and you will be able to download weekly meal plans and recipes. I have also given you a sample week to try.

* Before you buy food always read the label. Be awake to the tricky words used for sugar (maltodextrin, corn syrup, and most words ending in -ose) and the use of numbers for artificial flavours, colours and preservatives. If too many foreign ingredients are listed, or the product has a long shelf-life, don't buy it!

	ENJOY ✓	AVOID ✗
FRUIT—contain essential enzymes and vital nutrients which support the detox process.		
• Limit fruit intake to 3 serves/day due to their sugar content • Choose SLOW fruit where possible	All fresh fruit except bananas (high sugar)	Bananas, dried and tinned fruits
VEGETABLES—are a crucial part of any diet. They are alkalising and a great source of fibre, antioxidants, vitamins and phytonutrients. All support detoxing.		
• Have as many serves of vegetables and salad greens as you wish; at least 4 cups of salad and 3 cups of vegetables per day • Do not microwave or fry vegetables. • Choose SLOW vegetables if possible.	All vegetables and salad greens except those mentioned to avoid	Potatoes, pickled, tinned or frozen vegetables
PROTEINS—are the cell's building blocks. It is critical to build and maintain muscle mass, and boost your metabolism.		
• Choose lean protein sources (organic and free-range where possible) and try to make one serve a vegetarian option. • Include 1 serve at each meal (1 serve = the size and thickness of the palm of your hand). • Do not fry or barbeque meats.	Beans, chicken, chickpea, eggs, fish, kangaroo, lamb, lentils, soy beans, tempeh, tofu, turkey, veal	Bacon, beef, cured meats, deli meats, flake, mince, oysters, pork, salami, sausages, shellfish, smoked fish, smoked meats, sword fish, tuna

	ENJOY	AVOID
DAIRY—contains calcium and iron and fat soluble vitamins. Dairy products from cows should be avoided while on the four–week Get Clean Get Lean program.	✓	✗
• Dairy alternatives may be used but limit to 1 serve/day. (1 serve = 1 glass milk product)	Unsweetened, organic soy, rice, nut or goat's milk. Plain yoghurt (soy or goat's is preferable)	Cheese, cow's milk, cream, ice cream, sweetened soy milk, sweetened yoghurt
CARBOHYDRATES—provide energy, fibre and a number of vitamins (namely B group) and minerals. Wheat should be avoided on the program and limit intake of other grains.	✓	✗
• Limit grains to a maximum of 1 serve/day. (1 serve = 30g) as they are low in the required detox nutrients and contribute to an acidic body. • Try to eat organic and wholegrain carbs.	Amaranth, brown rice, buckwheat, millet, oats, plain rice cakes, quinoa, spelt or rye bread	biscuits, cakes, chips, couscous, packaged cereals, packaged muesli bars, all pastas, pastry, pizza, processed oats, triticale, wheat (including bread) etc.
NUTS, SEEDS & OILS—are a good source of protein, fibre and nutrients required for the detox process.	✓	✗
• Limit nuts and seeds to 2 serves/day. (1 serve = ¼ cup) • Limit oils to a maximum of 2 tablespoons/day. • Try to eat raw and organic where possible and use cold pressed oils. • Include flaxseed oil as it contains omega-3 fatty acids in the form of ALA (alpha linolenic acid) and cancer fighting lignans.	All raw nuts except peanuts, all seeds in small quantities, LSA mix, lecithin, cold pressed oils (olive, walnut, sesame, flax, coconut)	Peanuts, roasted or salted nuts. Peanut oil, most vegetable oils, canola oil, peanut butter.
HERBS, SPICES & CONDIMENTS—are a good way to flavour food and many have health promoting properties.	✓	✗
• Avoid table salt and any commercially prepared dressings and condiments.	Garlic, home-made dressings, home-made guacamole and hummus, organic tamari, tahini, sea salt etc.	Table salt and any commercially prepared dressings and condiments (tomato sauce, sweet chili sauce, soy sauce etc.)

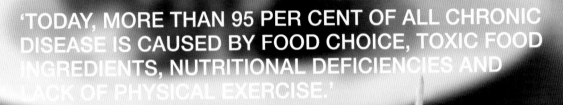

'TODAY, MORE THAN 95 PER CENT OF ALL CHRONIC DISEASE IS CAUSED BY FOOD CHOICE, TOXIC FOOD INGREDIENTS, NUTRITIONAL DEFICIENCIES AND LACK OF PHYSICAL EXERCISE.'

Mike Adams

SLOW FOOD

S is for seasonal
L is for LOCAL
O is for organic
W is for whole

Enjoy a nice variety of SLOW foods eaten, you guessed it ... slowly!

HOW TO COOK CLEAN FOOD AND KEEP IT CLEAN?

I went to boarding school for my senior years in high school, and I am sure the mantra by the kitchen staff was to keep us full on the smallest budget possible. To this day, I cannot eat white bread or potato, in any shape or form. Bread was the staple at every single meal and we could eat as much of it as we wanted. And potoes were dumped on our plates in salty, buttery mountains of sin. The vegies were cooked within an inch of their life and the meat was generally over-cooked too. Come to think of it, there was always a lot of white on our plates, and not so much colour, unless you count the tomato sauce. For someone who grew up on a farm with fresh fruit and vegetables every day and a mum who could cook as well as any budding chef, this was a major transition for me. Thankfully, I was on a special diet due to my hernia—although there wasn't too much special about it. Generally a really dry piece of fish with over-steamed vegies. Guess what I filled up on—potatoes and bread!

There comes a point in your life where you realise you can't go another day eating water-logged or over-cooked vegetables. And that potato, whether mashed, boiled, fried, or roasted, cannot be the main food on your plate. Jamie Oliver, where were you back in the 1980s?

We have all come a long way since then, and now understand, thanks to the good work of people like Jamie Oliver, that food is best when treated lovingly and cooked lightly. The less cooked your food, the more alive it will be. High heat denatures a lot of the enzymes present in food. And cooking in a big bath of water leaches the water soluble vitamins from the food. While you are on the Get Clean program try to eat at least 50 per cent of your food in its raw state: lots of salads, seeds, nuts and some fresh fruit. Remember to chew your food thoroughly so it is easily digested.

Some food, especially meat and starchy vegetables, are actually better if they are cooked. (although I am partial to a good sashimi). Cooking can break down some of the proteins or starches so they are easily digested in your body, as well as make the food more palatable. There is a clean way to cook your food, and a dirty way to destroy your food.

I've outlined the clean cooking methods on the next page. I won't dwell on the negative, however the dirtiest and most toxic ways you can cook your food are:

FRYING—Or you could just get a syringe and inject your food with copious amounts of oil. Even if you are using the best and purest oil on the planet, the high temp will break-down the fat chains and give off trans fats.

MICROWAVING—I know, this is a quick way of cooking, however it is also a quick way of stripping your food of any nutritional value and adding quite a few toxins. Studies show up to 97 per cent of the nutritional value of food is lost when microwaved.

BOILING—This isn't the worst way to cook your foods if you are going to do it quickly, however most of us throw things in boiling water and leave it for way too long. Steaming is a better option, or poaching in a small amount of water.

> When you cook your vegetables in water, save the water and drink as a tea or use as stock for soups and sauces. Notice the water has a colour to it; that indicates that some of the beneficial phytochemicals have leached out of the vegetable and into the water during the cooking process. That cooking water is now loaded with goodness. Pop it in your body, not down the sink.

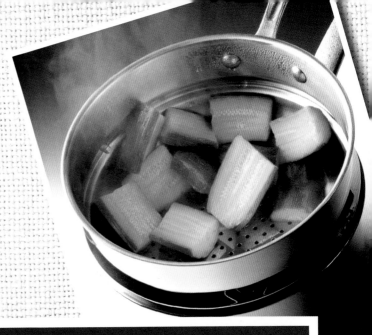

FIVE TIPS FOR CLEAN COOKING

In general, this is a gentle way of cooking food that enhances its nutritional value rather than taking it away. These include:

1 Steaming—This is a super healthy way to cook all food, from fish and chicken to vegetables. It retains most of the nutritional value of the food without the need to add fat. There are several ways to steam your food, from the bamboo steamer used in Asian cooking, to a double saucepan. You suspend the steamer over a pot of boiling water and the steam actually cooks the food. The food doesn't touch the water, so there is less chance of losing water soluble vitamins. This method is also quick.

2 Blanching—I love cooking asparagus and broccoli using this method. You dunk the food in boiling water for a short time—just enough to soften it slightly—then put the food in icy cold water. This stops the cooking process and leaves you with brightly coloured, just crisp vegetables.

3 Stir-frying—I love this way of cooking too. In a fry pan or wok, add a small amount of cold-pressed oil (olive or coconut) and over a medium heat toss your food through the heat. Keep your food moving so it cooks through evenly.

4 Grilling—This is a great way to cook meat as it allows the fat to drain away. If you are grilling vegetables, give them a light coting of olive oil so they don't dry out and become cardboard-like.

5 Baking/Roasting—Just because you are eating clean doesn't mean you have to go without your Sunday roast. Rather than have your food sitting in a pool of oil, set you meat up on a rack over water - the steam from the water keeps the meat moist. And before putting your vegetables in the oven, coat them lightly with olive oil and then roast them in the oven. In the recipe section there are some great clean cake and biscuit recipes you can try as well.

SUPPLEMENTS

Generally if you eat well you don't need to take supplements, although the nutrients in food aren't what they used to be and most of us are deficient in something. Zinc is definitely one of those nutrients. Also, with the level of toxicity in our diet and lifestyle, a probiotic can be really helpful, especially if you've been on medication (antibiotics) or suffer from bloating. And, of course, a good fish oil since we tend to have too much Ω6 and not enough Ω3.

The other supplement I swear by is a glutathione supplement called Cellgevity. It is one of the few supplements with a proprietary blend that encourages your cells to produce the glutathione as opposed to just supplementing. Glutathione supplements in the past have been unstable since they are broken down in the gut and don't make it to your cells where they are needed, so this particular formula is one I recommend.

While you are on the Get Clean program, having a supplement to support your liver while you are detoxing is a good idea. Milk thistle is great, plus it has an antioxidant and free radical scavenging action, making it especially beneficial.

You may have heard of Alpha Lipoic Acid (also known as lipoic acid, thioctic acid, or ALA)? It is one of the good fatty acids produced in every one of your cells. Its main functions is to help convert glucose (blood sugar) into energy. ALA is also an antioxidant. What's special about ALA is that it is both water and fat soluble. Scientists believe that ALA operates in conjunction with vitamins C and E, and the antioxidant glutathione, recycling them when they're used up. Without making too fine a point about it, Cellgevity also contains ALA, milk thistle and a few other goodies so it is great value for money.

The non-essential amino acid L-glutamine can be a great help while your insulin and blood sugar are rebalancing, especially if you are fighting sugar or carb cravings. Aside from reducing cravings, it:

- reduces fatigue
- improves endurance during exercise
- supports the liver and colon
- strengthens your immune system
- enhances memory and concentration

It's best taken on an empty stomach and is often added to many detox formulations. Before taking any supplements you should consult your health care professional first.

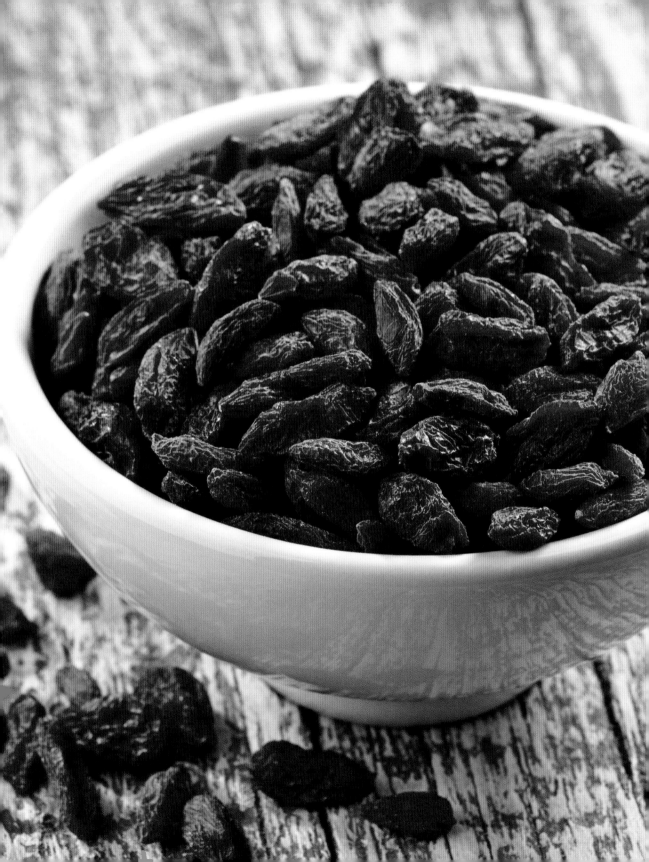

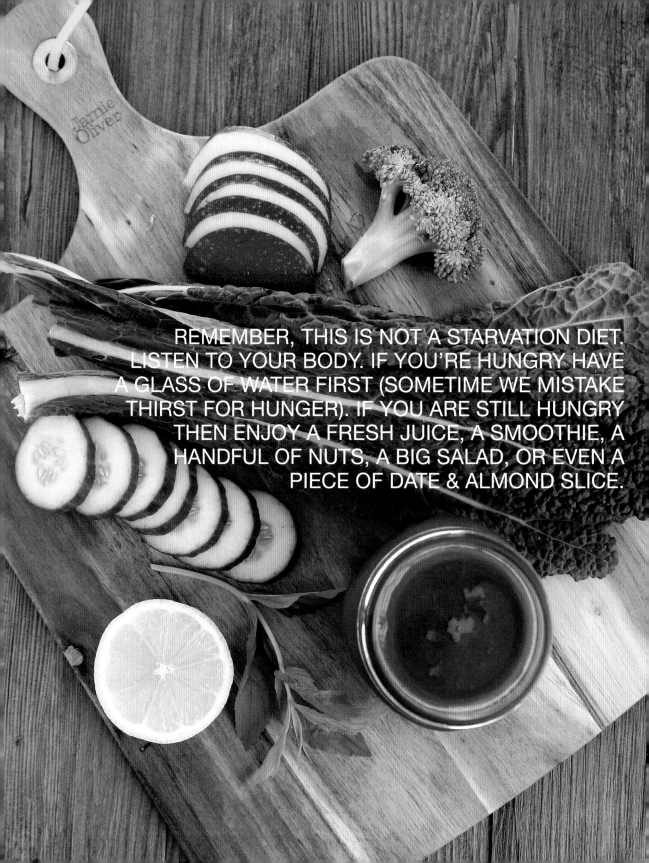

REMEMBER, THIS IS NOT A STARVATION DIET. LISTEN TO YOUR BODY. IF YOU'RE HUNGRY HAVE A GLASS OF WATER FIRST (SOMETIME WE MISTAKE THIRST FOR HUNGER). IF YOU ARE STILL HUNGRY THEN ENJOY A FRESH JUICE, A SMOOTHIE, A HANDFUL OF NUTS, A BIG SALAD, OR EVEN A PIECE OF DATE & ALMOND SLICE.

GO

So now you have a good understanding of nutrition, you know what foods to enjoy and what to avoid. You've cleaned your cupboards and stocked up on clean food. You've got your cooking basics down-pat. I think you're ready to get clean and get lean. The only thing left now is to do it! For the next 28 days you are going to treat your body like the temple it is. I should warn you, some days will be tough, but worth it. You won't know yourself at the end of the program. You are going to be one vital, vibrant, full of energy person, ready to take on anything life throws at you.

And then once you're clean and lean there will be no going back. You won't want to. Because you'll know what it is like to have clear skin, no bloats or headaches, you'll have lost weight, you'll be sleeping better, you'll listen to and hear your body telling you things, and your tastes will have changed. That's when you'll adopt the Low HI way of eating (Step 2). Not a diet, not a fad, just a great way of eating to stay healthy and vital for life. But for now LETS GET CLEAN GET LEAN.

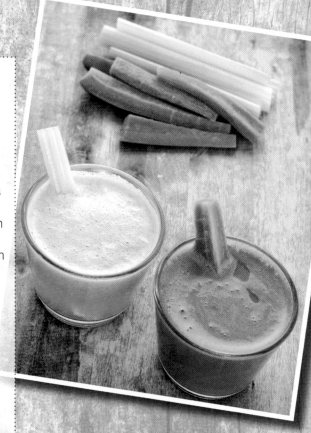

A quick recap:

✓ dry body brush before jumping into the shower

✓ look in the mirror and like what you see (smile)

✓ finish shower with the water on cold for 30 seconds

✓ have apple cider vinegar before breakfast and lunch

✓ if you're taking supplements remember to take them

✓ drink eight glasses of water

✓ eat only what's on the 'allowed list'

✓ exercise for at least 30 minutes

✓ take time-out to breathe

✓ book a spa or massage treatment

SEVEN DAYS SAMPLE GET CLEAN GET LEAN EATING PLAN

This seven-day plan is simply a guide to help you out until you get in the groove of creating your own meal plans. This is a BIG step in the education process of what you should eat rather than someone spoon-feeding you (pun intended) every day. You'll learn to listen to your body and make proper decisions for you and your health like the smart individual you are. Where there is an asterisk (*) it means the recipe is at the back of the book.

	Monday	Tuesday	Wednesday
BREAKFAST	Poached egg on rye or whole grain toast Avocado spread (or olive oil) Spinach	Home-made Granola* 1 cup berries	2 Egg Green Omlette* (no dairy; use olive oil) Serve with tomato and mushrooms
SNACK	1 piece fruit Handful of nuts	Green Juice*	Raw Date and Almond Slice*
LUNCH	BIG salad with lean meat (chicken, beef or tuna) Lots of green vegetables and a vinegarette dressing	Detox Garden Salad with Wasabi Dressing*	Freestyle salad with any colourful veggies, avocado and Best Zesty Dressing*
SNACK	Kamalaya Detox Juice*	Toss frozen berries, a sliced banana and 2 tablespoons chia seeds in a covered glass container and let it sit in the refrigerator overnight.	1 piece fruit Handful of nuts
DINNER	Protein smoothie	Lean protein and 75 per cent vegetables (some raw, some cooked)	Eggplant Moussaka on Spinach with Roasted Tomato sauce*

EVERY DAY: Don't forget to drink 8 glasses of water (and enjoy herbal teas), and remember to take your supplements.

Do not beat yourself up if you stray and have sugar or a glass of wine. You're only human. Get straight back on the bike (so to speak) and keep going forward. Some days will be better than others. Just remember WHY you are doing this, WHAT is your goal, and HOW are you going to reward yourself at the end.

Thursday	Friday	Saturday	Sunday
Home-made Granola* 1 cup berries	Scrambled eggs (no dairy; use olive oil) Spinach, tomato and mushrooms	Oats with a sprinkle of seeds and nuts. ½ cup strawberries	2 Egg Green Omlette* (no dairy; use olive oil) Serve with tomato and mushrooms
Green Juice*	1 piece fruit Handful of nuts	1 piece fruit Handful of nuts	Kamalaya Detox Juice*
Asian Style Thai Pumpkin Soup*	Superfood Black Bean and Quinoa Salad*	BIG salad with lean meat (chicken, beef or tuna) Lots of green vegetables and a vinegarette dressing	Asian-style Thai Pumpkin Soup*
Toss frozen berries, a sliced banana and 2 tablespoons chia seeds in a covered glass container and let it sit in the refrigerator over-night.	Green juice	Hummus and vegetables	Raw Date & Almond Slice*
Som Tam*	Lean protein and 75 per cent vegetables (some raw, some cooked)	Prawn Rice Paper Rolls*	Poached Sea Bass with Soya and Thai Seafood Sauce*

CREATE YOUR OWN SEVEN DAY GET CLEAN GET LEAN EATING PLAN

P lanning your meals is a really good habit to get into, and it takes the pressure off 'what am I going to make for dinner'? It also takes care of your shopping list and ensures you are eating a balanced diet. Buy only want you plan to eat, and only from the 'enjoy' list.

	Monday	Tuesday	Wednesday
BREAKFAST			
SNACK			
LUNCH			
SNACK			
DINNER			

EVERY DAY: Don't forget to drink 8 glasses of water (and enjoy herbal teas), and remember to take your supplements.

TREAT YOURSELF TO A BATH

An epsom salts bath is not only great for muscle soreness, but also draws impurities out of your body. Simply add two cups of epsom salts, two cups baking soda, and 5–10 drops of your favorite essential oils to a warm bath and soak, and viola! The salts draw the toxins from your body and the baking soda neutralises acids on the skin, helping dissolve exterior toxins like oil and perspiration. This bath cleanses both inside and out! Add some candles and music if you want to create a soothing spa ambience. Experts say to soak for 20 minutes to allow the epsom salts (magnesium sulfate) to draw the toxins out, however no more than 20 minutes as you may start re-absorbing the impurities.

Thursday	Friday	Saturday	Sunday

KEEPING TRACK OF HOW YOU FEEL

Week	Day 1	Day 2	Day 3	Day 4	Day 5	Day 6	Day 7
1							
2							
3							
4							

If you feel inclined, keep a journal of how you feel each day. And then reflect back once you hit day 28. You can download this form from krisabbey.com

HIGH FIVES ...

But low(er) blood sugar, blood pressure, cholesterol and weight! Well done to you; and how do you feel? Don't forget to reward yourself with whatever your intention was at the start of the program. You deserve to be proud of yourself and what you have done for you.

Enjoy how great you feel, and get ready to continue on this path of good, clean health and vitality (although not quite as rigid). You are ready to enjoy the Low HI way of eating. Put simply, eating a wonderful array of tasty foods that have had Low Human Intervention ... that is, food that is fresh, natural and not made in a manufacturing plant with synthetic ingredients.

NOTES

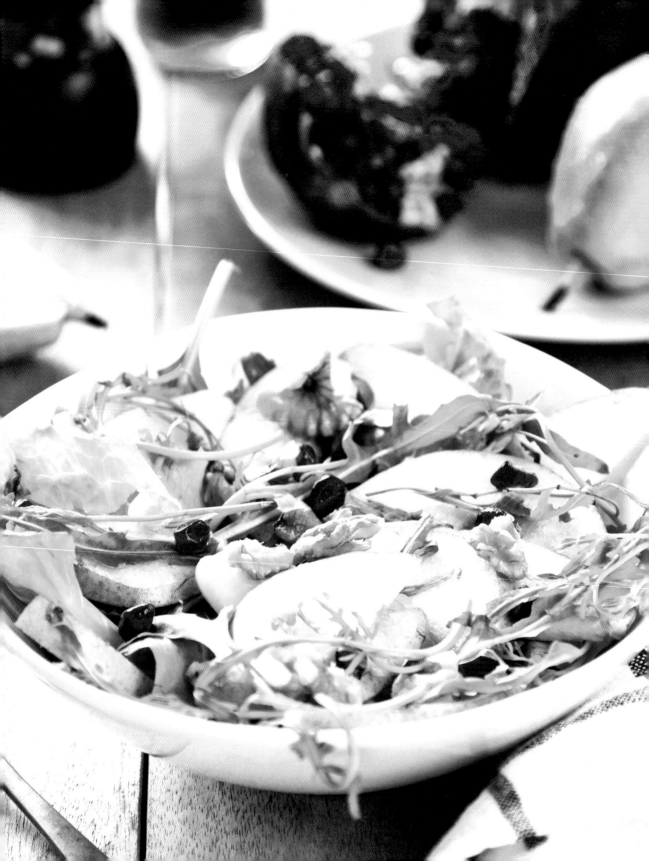

STEP 2
The LOW HI
way of eating

'Don't eat anything your great-great grandmother wouldn't recognise as food. There are a great many food-like items in the supermarket your ancestors wouldn't recognise as food ... stay away from these.' Michael Pollan

WHAT IS LOW HI?

Low HI is a term I coined when I was trying to think up the '30 second elevator pitch' of what is the most nutritious way to eat? I get that question a lot.

Thinking about what is the most nutritious way of eating, I started going through what I know, what I have experienced, and what I see in the older people around me who are vital and healthy compared to those the same age who are not. I concluded it is eating real food as fresh as possible. It's eating real food that hasn't had chemicals added to it, it is eating real food that hasn't been poured out of a box or that has been sitting in your fridge or pantry for months. It is food that comes form Mother Earth, and not man-made. It is actually eating foods that have had low human intervention, or Low HI.

If you look at all the lifestyle-related illnesses and where they stem from—it is poor diet. More specifically, eating a highly processed diet containing foods with a lot of additives. If you were to eat natural foods, or foods that haven't been so denatured it is hard to recognise their original form (seriously, does a wheat flake even resemble a grain of wheat?), I can guarantee you would be healthier, our country would be healthier. Heck, I'm going to go out on a limb and say the whole world would be healthier. Big call, but ample evidence to back it up.

In a large, newly published study of more than 6200 Americans, researchers from Johns Hopkins and other universities found that four lifestyle behaviours were associated with reducing the risk of lifestyle related diseases: namely, lower incidence of calcium deposits in coronary arteries (calcium build-up increases heart attack risk) and lower rates of cardiovascular events like heart attacks and angina (chest pain). In fact, the study showed a reduced risk of death from all causes by 80 per cent. You'll never guess what the four factors were:

THE FOUR LIFESTYLE FACTORS FOR LIVING LONGER AND BETTER WERE:

1. Not smoking
2. Keeping a normal weight
3. Exercising regularly—150 minutes or more of moderately intense physical activity per week, or 75 minutes or more of vigorous activity per week.
4. Eating a healthy diet—high in vegetables, legumes, fruits, nuts, whole grains, and fish, and low in meat, full-fat dairy, poultry, and other saturated-fat-rich foods.

And there it is. I'm sure that study cost a lot of money to do, but unfortunately these days common sense needs to be proven by science before people will accept it.

The days of prepackaged low-fat high-carb food have passed. We are about to experience a real food revolution, or at least we can start one!

The Low HI way of eating is so simple I can summarise it in less than one page. Now that your body is clean and lean, you want to continue those habits and enjoy healthy eating for life.

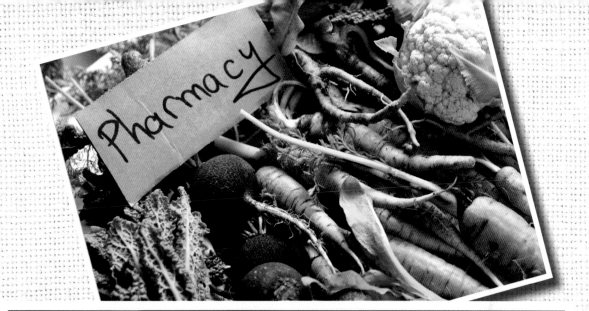

PRINCIPLES TO EATING LOW HI

You've actually been eating this way for the last 28 days on the Get Clean Get Lean program, however now you can now relax a little and let a few things creep in. If you like a bit of cheese or fancy a piece of steak, now is the time to enjoy. Think about your choices, and make the right one. For example, instead of instant pasta in a box, get fresh pasta without all the preservatives.

* Buy seasonal, local (preferrably organic) and whole fruit and vegetables.
* Buy cold-pressed oils not cheap vegetable oil blends.
* Choose lean cuts of meat and eat processed meats such as bacon very very rarely.
* Choose raw, unsalted nuts not roasted, salted, or suagr-coated ones.
* Avoid any food that can sit on a pantry shelf for long periods (except legumes and wholegrains).
* Eat the real version of the food not the man-made one (cheese in a can, what is that?).
* If it comes in a box, and has words like 'quick', 'instant' or 'baked not fried' it's High HI.
* Use natural flavours on food such as fresh herbs and spices over artificial ones.
* Make your own sauces and dressings rather than commercial toxic ones.
* Enjoy fresh baked bread that is dark and heavy not light white loaves that come in plastic wrappers.
* Learn to bake using natural sweetners and wheat-free flour alternatives.
* Stay away from artificial sweetners, soft drink and especially diet soft drinks.
* Make your own fresh juices rather than buying commercial ones (even the no added sugar ones are high in sugar). Add vegetables too so the natural sugar content isn't as high.
* Avoid all commercial cakes, baked goods and lollies.
* Don't eat food that contains trans fat.
* Make your own savoury snacks—you love chips, home-made in a good oil is a healthier option.
* And stop being lazy, quit buying snack foods in packets for you and your kids' lunch boxes. Don't pass your sugar addiction onto them. They will eat what you give them to eat and develop a taste for it.

LOW-FAT IS A BIG FAT LIE

by Dr Dwight Lundell, MD

What you are about to read requires an open mind. You have to look at facts instead of massive advertising and failed, faulty theories. You almost have to disregard a lot of what you thought was true about food and weight loss (that is, prior to reading this book!). Are you ready?

Fact: From 1900 to 1980, obesity rates in the US remained stable at 14 per cent to 15 per cent of the population. Since 1980, however, obesity rates have skyrocketed. Today, 65 per cent of the population is overweight or obese. This spike is directly linked to the US Department of Agriculture's creation of the food pyramid, advocating 11 daily servings of grains and cereals. This is not a coincidence.

For most of my 25-year medical career and 5,000 heart surgeries, I accepted low-fat dieting theories. I also believed the theory that dietary cholesterol was a primary cause of heart disease. But as heart disease continued to soar, year after year, my doubts increased.

I treated thousands of patients after they became ill. The question that haunted me was what was causing heart disease, obesity and diabetes in the first place? As I examined the data, it was clear that these conditions spiked in the 1980s, then continued to climb.

Study after study has demonstrated the negative effects of consuming a grain-based, low-fat, high-sugar diet. There is no credible evidence to suggest that a low-fat diet equals a lower incidence of heart disease and obesity. In fact, all the evidence proves otherwise. The low-fat and cholesterol theories are based on incomplete science.

'We are what we eat' is a common saying. But it is not quite accurate. Instead of focusing on what we put inside our bodies, we should focus on how our bodies metabolise the food we put there. How we metabolise low-fat, high-sugar and grain-based food is clearly reflected in our growing rates of obesity and heart disease. More people develop heart disease today than ever before, and at an earlier age. Every 34 seconds, a person in the US loses their life to a heart attack. That's 2500 people a day.

The National Institutes of Health, the National Cholesterol Education Program, the American Heart Association, the US Department of Agriculture and a host of other medical organisations continue to advocate a low-fat diet and statin medications to reduce cholesterol. These organisations are wrong, but to admit it threatens their bottom line.

You don't have time to wait for the government, the medical community and food manufacturers to admit their mistake. If you have faithfully followed their mistaken regime, you can stop blaming yourself for excess pounds and ill health. Your life and your health happens now and it's in your control. Read that bit again!

The low-fat and cholesterol theories are firmly planted in our consciousness. From the advice of our physicians, to the TV ads for statin drugs, to the grocery store aisles packed with low-fat foods, these faulty theories are reinforced at every turn. Their powerful marketing may be persuasive, but it is not scientific fact.

REAL FOOD (OR LOW HI)

The first step you should take to improving your health is to return to the diet of your grandparents in the days before governments and food manufacturers declared war on fat and real food to fit faulty theories. Your grandparents were not afraid to drink real milk and eat eggs, butter and red meat.

I am not advocating these foods in large quantities. But their elimination from our diet—in favour of low-fat, high-sugar, grain-based foods—has resulted in inflammation and staggering rates of obesity.

Packaged low-fat foods created for shelf life—not human life—never touched your grandparents' plates. Hydrogenated omega-6 vegetable oils and margarine were not even invented. For your grandparents, sugar was a treat reserved for special occasions. Now it is a daily staple.

Drug companies have done a magnificent job convincing us that we cannot get well without medication. This is not true. Your body is a tremendous, self-healing organism. When you consume real food and essential nutrients, it will respond and flourish.

Packaged low-fat foods filled with sugar and omega-6 oils strongly contribute to inflammation. This is the true cause of heart disease, diabetes and a host of other diseases. There is no better time than now to understand how the faulty cholesterol theory has created an epidemic of inflammation and what you can do about it. You only have one heart. Keeping it healthy is not nearly as difficult as you might think.

ABOUT THE AUTHOR

Dr Dwight Lundell is the past Chief of Staff and Chief of Surgery at Banner Heart Hospital, Mesa, Arizona. He is the founder of the Healthy Humans Foundation and Chief Medical Advisor for Asantae. In 2003, he made the most difficult decision of his 25-year surgical career. As traditional medicine continued to chase the cholesterol theory of heart disease, he closed his surgical practice and devoted the rest of his life to speaking the truth—that inflammation causes heart disease. By lowering inflammation, heart disease has a cure.

Dr Lundell is the author of the worldwide bestselling book, *The Great Cholesterol Lie*, a revealing look at heart disease and the faulty theories of low-fat diets and cholesterol. In this book, he also reveals his clinically-tested recommendations for lowering inflammation to prevent and reverse heart disease.

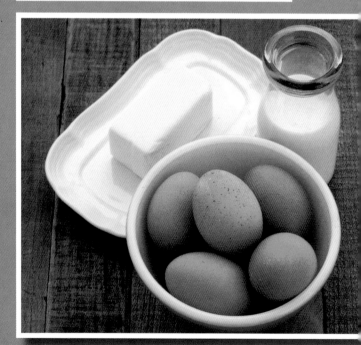

WHAT'S IN SEASON

SUMMER		AUTUMN	
FRUIT	**VEGETABLES**	**FRUIT**	**VEGETABLES**
Avocadoes	Asparagus	Apples	Asian greens
Apricots	Beans—green, flat,	Bananas	Avocados
Bananas	butter	Berries	Beetroot
Berries—blackberries,	Capsicum	Grapes	Broccoli
blueberries, raspberries	Celery	Kiwifruit	Brussels sprouts
strawberries, cherries	Chillies	Lemons	Cabbage
Figs	Cucumber	Limes	Carrots
Grapes	Eggplant	Mandarin	Cauliflower
Limes	Lettuce	Nashi	Celery
Lychees	Okra	Oranges	Eggplant
Mangoes	Peas	Papaya	Fennel
Melons	Potatoes	Passionfruit	Garlic
Nectarines	Radish	Pears	Ginger
Oranges—Valencia	Sweet corn	Plums	Leeks
Papaya	Tomatoes	Pomegranate	Lettuce
Passionfruit	Watercress	Rhubarb	Mushrooms
Pawpaw	Zucchini	Tamarillo	Onions
Peaches			Parsnip
Pears—Williams			Peas
Pineapple			Potato
Plums			Pumpkin
			Spinach
			Swede
			Sweet corn
			Sweet potato
			Tomato
			Zucchini

Seasonal fruit and vegetables should make up about 50 per cent of your diet. The rest should come from lean sources of protein, good fats, and low GI carbs—remember our plate on page 28. Try to stick to that as much as you can.

WINTER		SPRING	
FRUIT	VEGETABLES	FRUIT	VEGETABLES
Apples—Fuji, Golden delicious, Granny Smith, Jonathans, Pink Lady	Artichoke	Apples—Pink Lady	Artichokes—globe
Avocados	Beetroot	Avocados	Asian greens
Bananas	Broad beans	Bananas	Asparagus
Grapefruit—Ruby Red	Brussels sprouts	Berries	Broad beans
Kiwifruit	Cabbage—red	Cherries	Beetroot
Lemons	Cauliflower	Grapefruit	Cucumber
Limes	Celeriac	Lemons	Cauliflower
Mandarins	Celery	Mandarins—Honey	Broccoli
Nashi Pears	Eggplants	Murcott	Carrots
Pineapple	Fennel	Mangoes	Cauliflower
Loquats	Leeks	Melons	Chillies
Rhubarb	Mushrooms	Rockmelon	Garlic—fresh
	Okra	Oranges—Valencia	Lettuce
	Parsnips	Papaya	Mushrooms
	Parsley	Pineapples	Onions—spring and shallots
	Pumpkins	Passionfruit	Peas
	Quinces	Pawpaw	Potatoes
	Rhubarb	Strawberries	Silverbeet
	Sweet potato		Sweetcorn
	Sweet corn		Spinach
	Silver beet		Tomatoes
	Spinach		Watercress
	Turnips		Zucchini and zucchini flowers
	Wild rocket		

THE JOURNEY TO YOUR PLATE

While fresh is best, many nutrients start degrading soon after the vegetable is picked. Therefore the longer they are stored, the fewer vitamins, minerals and antioxidants they will contain. For example, after being refrigerated for eight days, English spinach has lost 47 percent of its folate and 46 percent of its carotenes. And when you buy those strawberries out of season, ripened in a refrigerated shipping container as they made the trip from Colombia, remember that they don't have nearly the vitamins, antioxidants or tastiness that their summer cousins have.

By the time a vegetable gets to your dinner plate it has been:
* picked
* packed
* loaded onto trucks
* transported by road, rail or air
* sold at market
* delivered to the retailer
* stored
* unpacked
* sat on the shelf
* purchased by you
* sat in your fridge
* and then . . . finally used.
At the very least, this process can take days. But it can also be weeks or months!

Buying locally grown food also supports nearby farmers, and greatly reduces the energy and resources necessary to transport and store foods.
* Seasonal food means seeds germinate in the soil at the right time, meaning plants are naturally stronger and more resistant to disease. This gives better quality fruit and vegetables.
* Out-of-season food may be 'force grown' in artificial conditions, requiring more fertilisers. This can lead to watery, flavourless produce.
* Food left to ripen on the plant will contain more nutrients and have a better flavour than food that is harvested early and ripened artificially.
* It's a fact that most fruit and vegetables start to lose their flavour and nutritional value as soon as they're picked.

Buying local, seasonal food guarantees you shorter times from paddock to plate. Out-of-season food may have been picked six or more weeks before you buy it. Doesn't sound too fresh or nutritious.

DRINK TO THAT

What you drink is very important and has a major impact on your body. Up to now we have been focussing on water, water and more water—to flush and hydrate. The aim is to keep toxins from your body and they creep in just as easily in your drinks as they do in your food. So, soft drinks (especially diet ones) are off limits. If you need some fizz, have plain sparkling mineral water (go for low sodium) and add flavour with a slice of lime and some mint leaves. Throw in a fake umbrella for full effect. Herbal teas are a great beverage as you get added health benefits (usually antioxidants) without added caffiene. And, of course. fresh juices and smoothies (especially of the veggie-based, green variety). Try to have one every day as they are a super health kick and a great toxic mop. The odd glass of wine (you know the drill—no more than two glasses in a week while detoxing, and then try to have no more than two glasses on say no more than three nights a week when you move onto eating low HI—think of the sugar!). But what about coffee?

I love my morning coffee and would be lost without it. I have a straight up long black. And you may have noticed that I allow you one cup (but not instant coffee) a day while on the detox. Do not add sugar and opt for black rather than adding milk (even if just while on detox). These rules apply to tea too. Coffee does have some antioxidants and minerals; however, its main clain to fame is the caffeine and the effects it has on your limbic system. It improves your focus, concentration, mood, mental alertness and even reduces muscle pain. It also helps with fat mobilisation, which is why athletes love it—it gives them a 'pick-up'—as well as helping them use fat as an energy source, sparing their glycogen stores.

Studies of Finnish and Swedish coffee drinkers found that two or three cups of coffee a day lowered the risk of developing Alzheimer's disease. And, similar results were found when US neuroscientists followed a group of coffee-drinking 65- to 88-year-olds who were just starting to show the first signs of memory loss. Those who drank about three cups of coffee a day avoided developing dementia.

Like many things though, more of a good thing is not always better. Caffeine is a stimulant so it isn't a great beverage if you're suffering stress, hypertension, or are having trouble sleeping. Try to avoid drinking coffee in the afternoon and, again, do not add sugar, cream or other nasties. Once you've had your coffee black, you'll start to appreciate the true taste of coffee—just be warned though, you do become a coffee snob!

CAFFEINE CONTENT

Freshly brewed coffee (250 mL cup*)	60–120 mg
Instant coffee (1 teaspoon)	60–80 mg
Black tea (250 mL cup)	10–50 mg
Energy drinks (e.g. Red Bull)	80 mg
Coca-cola (375 mL can)	36 mg
Milk chocolate (100 g bar)	20 mg

*Wide variation due to different brewing methods

Source: Australia New Zealand Food Authority (ANZFA)

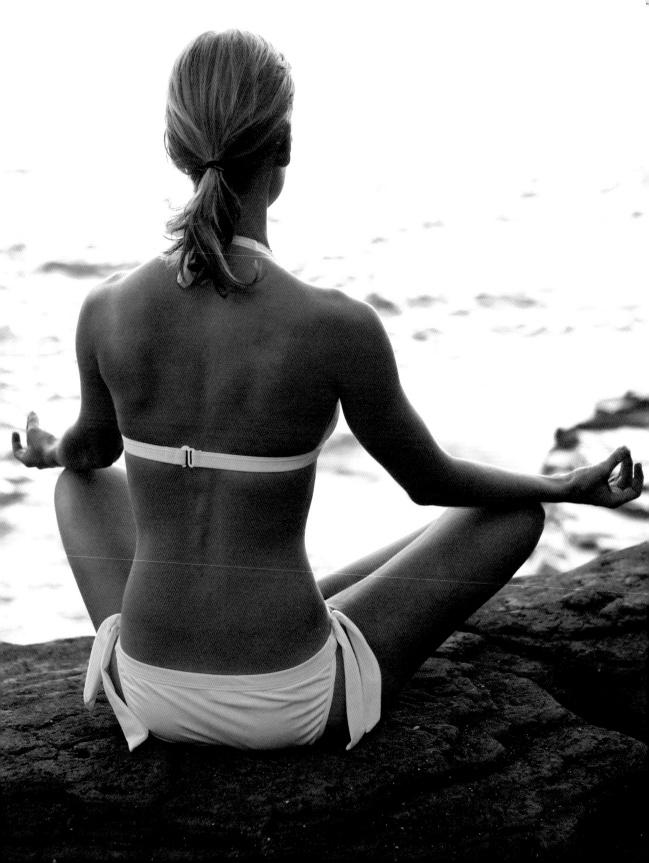

STEP 3

Enjoy Life | Age Well

Health and cheerfulness naturally beget each other.
Joseph Addison

HEALTH AND HAPPINESS

As we get older, and maybe wiser, we start to ask ourselves questions like 'Am I happy, do I love my job, could I be a better person, partner or parent?' All these questions crop up when you sit back and re-evaluate your life and where you are heading.

One of the main principles of Institute of Integrative Nutrition (IIN) is the concept of primary foods. Primary foods, or non-food sources of nourishment, are what really fuel us and go beyond the plate, nurturing us on a deeper level. The four main primary foods are:

❋   career
❋   relationships
❋   physical activity
❋   spirituality.

Can you remember being deeply in love? Everything is light and warm, colours are vivid, and life is full of joy. You float on air, and food becomes secondary. Now, recall a time you were depressed or experiencing low self-esteem—you were starving for primary food. No matter how much you ate, you never felt satisfied. The need for love, power, or mere acknowledgement drove the desire for excess food. Being happy and fulfilled plays a huge role in your health. Unhappiness, stress and poor-self esteem are detrimental to your health. Not just on a psychological level; they cause deep physiological issues as well. The exercise on the next page is a quick and simple way of seeing what areas in your life are lacking. Indentifying (and acknowledging) these allows you to do something about them. If there is an area in your life that is leaving you disatissfied, set some goals to change it. Your Circle of Life may take on a different shape each time you do it. That's the good thing, things can change. However, if you want change to happen you must change what you do or how you do it.

HAPPINESS

Deepak Chopra MD, world-renowned author, alternative medicine practitioner (and guru) says, 'Our entire reality and how we take care of ourselves is based on our sense of self. This includes the quality of our intention and attention to all matters. Health comes from connection. The origins of the word 'health' come from the word 'whole'. Health is wholeness, and when our sense of self is whole, we can finally achieve good health. Only 5 per cent of human genes are influenced solely by genetics. 95 per cent can be influenced by lifestyle choices and the state of our consciousness.'

And it's not just spiritual leaders who are pushing the happiness and wellbeing barrow. Political leaders including Nicolas Sarkozy and Barack Obama subscribe to the idea that measuring a nation's well-being by its economic output—its GDP per capita—is a policy dead-end. Mr David Cameron has been thinking along these lines for a while. Shortly after he became Tory leader in 2005, he said: 'Wellbeing can't be measured by money or traded in markets. It's about the beauty of our surroundings, the quality of our culture and, above all, the strength of our relationships. Improving our society's sense of wellbeing is, I believe, the central political challenge of our times.' He added: 'It's time we admitted that there's more to life than money and it's time we focused not just on GDP but on GWB—general wellbeing.'

Happiness and fulfillment play a major role in your health and consequently how you age. The secret to longevity is simple: nourish yourself with your primary foods, eat a healthy Low HI diet, enjoy exercise, reduce stress, and continue to challenge yourself to evolve. Make an effort in all of these areas and see the turn your life takes.

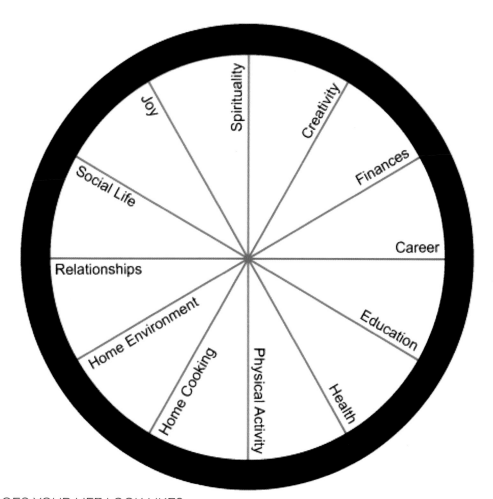

WHAT DOES YOUR LIFE LOOK LIKE?

Discover which primary foods you are missing, and how to infuse joy and satisfaction into your life.

1. Place a dot on the line in each category to indicate your level of satisfaction within each area. Place a dot at the center of the circle to indicate dissatisfaction, or on the periphery to indicate satisfaction. Most people fall somewhere in between (see example).

2. Connect the dots to see your Circle of Life.

3. Identify imbalances. Determine where to spend more time and energy to create balance.

© Integrative Nutrition | Kris Abbey

Example

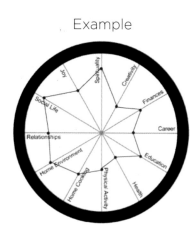

WHAT IS STRESS?

S tress is a prehistoric response that is rooted in a gland in your brain called the hypothalamus. An external trigger, or stressor, such as a tight deadline, stimulates the release of chemicals that tell your body to either stand and fight, or to run for its life.

When this happens, blood is withdrawn from your brain and stomach and sent to your larger muscle groups, adrenalin is released into your blood, your heart and lungs work harder, your eyes dilate, your skin sweats, the level of fats, cholesterol and sugar in your bloodstream increases, your stomach secretes more acid, your immune system slows down and your thinking shifts to a more black-and-white, survivalist mode.

Unfortunately, all this activity is not terribly useful in today's world. The stress response was designed to protect our hunter gatherer ancestors from immediate danger, such as predators. It was not designed for the more unrelenting stressors in modern life, like job insecurity, an unforgiving boss or information overload. 'Physiologically, we haven't evolved to live in the modern environment,' says Annie Ross, a psychologist who runs the stress management consultancy Health Initiatives, 'and that's why there is a stress epidemic causing so much illness, particularly mental illness.'

A recent guide to dealing with workplace stress called 'Stress: The Spice of Life or the Kiss of Death?' explores the paradox that, when we feel in control, stress becomes the spice of life, a challenge instead of a threat. Yet when we lack this crucial sense of control, stress can spell crisis.

A healthy level of stress helps us be productive, motivated and stimulated. It induces 'cortex thinking', or high-level, critical thinking that allows us to make good decisions. According to Ross, the danger lies in not turning this stress response off. 'When we experience stress, our body is releasing chemicals designed for fight or flight,

but instead of punching the boss or running out of the room, we sit quietly at our computers.'

If our stress has no outlet over time, our stress response can become hyperactive. This creates 'limbic thinking', or low-level thinking that involves losing the ability to process information clearly and rationally. We start overreacting to small things and we make bad decisions. This is when stress starts to affect work performance, health and relationships. It becomes a vicious cycle as we become exhausted, feel de-motivated and are less likely to behave in a way that would help us release stress, like exercising, seeing friends or just indulging ourselves with a warm bath and some candles.

NICE NOT NEGATIVE

Harville Hendrix PhD, world-renowned relationship expert and author of *Getting the Love You Want: Negativity is the Disease of the Human Race*, says 'Neuroscience has proven that negativity is our default stance as a means of self-preservation (think early humans needing to be prepared for worst-case scenarios), but we can change that by consciously focusing on the positive. The "put-down" is the biggest toxin of the human race. Next time you're in disagreement with your partner, ask yourself if the way you are speaking is putting them down or lifting them up?'

BEHAVIOURAL	PSYCHOLOGICAL/EMOTIONAL	PHYSICAL
Increased intake of cigarettes, alcohol, drugs or food	Increased anxiety	Headaches
Declining work performance	Depression	Insomnia
Poor relationships	Irritability	Persistent indigestion
Insomnia	Aggression	Constipation or diarrhoea
Avoiding situations or people	Mood swings	Regular colds and flu (particularly on holidays)
Low sex drive		Chronic tiredness
Negativity		Skin rashes
		Palpitations
		Excessive sweating
		Tight throat
		Chest pain
		Stomach pain
		Neck or back pain

This table shows common signs of negative stress.

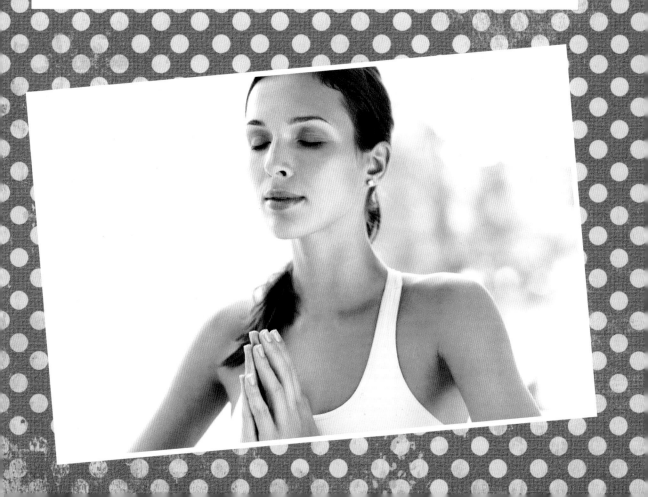

According to Dr Cate Howell and Dr Michele Murphy, authors of *Release Your Worries*, there are many simple strategies you can use to regain balance in your life and feel less stressed. The following 10 tips are from their book:

1 RELAXATION

Relaxation means different things to different people. Relaxation can include slow breathing techniques or meditation, or active relaxation such as sport or exercise. Think about what you find relaxing and build it into your day. Some people relax by reading, having a massage or a hot bath, engaging in a hobby, or getting in touch with nature by taking a walk in the park.

2 DO THINGS YOU VALUE

We live in complex times and lead increasingly busy and demanding lives. We want more and more, but know we can't have it all, at least not all at the same time! With so much competing for our attention, we need to have clear priorities to be able to choose how we spend our precious time and energy. What have been the most rewarding parts of your life so far? What has brought you joy? What has inspired you and what gives you meaning? The answers to these questions should lead you to understand what you value the most. If you prioritise these areas, you may feel less stressed as you're no longer spreading yourself too thin.

3 CONNECT WITH FRIENDS

Good social support can be a great buffer against stress, so surround yourself with people who know how to relax and have fun.

4 BE IN THE MOMENT

A new movement known as 'mindfulness' emphasises the importance of being fully present at any given moment. By fully engaging in the present, you are less likely to worry about the past or future. You can also decrease your stress levels by choosing to take action in the present moment, whereas you have less control over the past or the future.

5 USE HUMOUR

Simple ways to de-stress using humour include watching a favourite comedy show, listening to what little kids say, and trying to see the funny side of a situation.

6 A HEALTHY LIFESTYLE

Eating healthy foods and getting adequate sleep and regular exercise all assist in helping you cope with daily stressors.

7 CHALLENGE YOUR NEGATIVE THOUGHTS

Most people have automatic thinking habits that can be unhelpful—habits such as 'all or nothing' thinking, such as 'If I don't get full marks in this test, I'm a failure'. You need to substitute these unhelpful thinking patterns with more helpful and realistic thoughts, such as 'I am an intelligent and valuable person, regardless of my test mark'.

8 LEARN TO SAY NO

We often worry that people will not like us, or approve of us, if we don't agree to do what they want. It's OK to say no, or to decline invitations to do things for others that will be at the expense of yourself. Most people will appreciate your clear boundaries and honesty.

9 PRIORITISE YOURSELF

You won't be of use to anyone if you are stressed to the point that you burn out. Prioritise your own self-care to ensure you are able to take care of your loved ones.

10 SELF COMPASSION

Take comfort in the knowledge that everyone feels stressed at some time and we are all in this together. If you compare yourself to others and find yourself lacking, remember that you are not necessarily privy to the whole picture. It is important to be kind and encouraging to yourself for all your efforts, regardless of the outcome.

SLEEP AND RELAXATION

One in three adults experience sleep problems during their life, often as a result of stress. Lack of sleep inhibits your concentration and slows your reaction time during waking hours, leading to reduced productivity and even accidents. It is important to break this cycle. Here's a few tips how:

* Develop a nightly routine to condition your body to recognise the cues for winding down and preparing for sleep.
* Try to go to bed and get up at the same time each day.
* Keep your bed as a place for sleep and sex, not for worrying. You may need to write down a list of your worries before going to bed.
* Avoid rich and spicy foods within three hours of going to bed.
* Limit coffee and tea to three cups a day and not within three hours of going to bed.
* Exercise during the day, but not within three hours of going to bed.
* Don't smoke, and keep your alcohol consumption within recommended limits. (For women, two standard drinks per day, with two alcohol-free days per week.)
* Avoid naps during the day.
* Try to avoid or minimise sleeping drugs, since these only address the symptom, not the underlying cause of the problem.
* Learn techniques for muscle relaxation, aromatherapy or meditation to help you relax and unwind.

INSANITY HAS BEEN DEFINED AS
REPEATING THE SAME ACTION AND
EXPECTING A DIFFERENT RESULT

SEVEN TIPS FOR SETTING AND ATTAINING GOALS

Things don't just happen, even though you closed your eyes and wished real hard as you blew out the candles on your cake. If you want some thing badly enough, make a plan to achieve it.

1 What do you desire? Write down exactly what you want. Be very specific. Describe it in sufficient detail to make it measurable. Just wanting to have lots of money or a new car is not enough. You need to be able to tell when you have what you want. Describe it as if you have it now.

2 Get organised. To be in control of your life, you need to be organised, with systems in place to help you move efficiently toward your goals and reduce stress.

3 Know how to prioritise. Learn how to put tasks in the correct order, from most important to least. Otherwise you may find yourself constantly busy, but not moving effectively toward your goals.

4 Be a visualiser. Channel the incredible power of your mind to actually see yourself and your life the way you want it to be. This is a great way to stay on track and reach your dreams.

5 Innovate and be creative. Cultivating the ability to go beyond the traditional ways you've done something can lead to powerful new solutions in many types of situations.

6 Focus on what you want. What you focus on is what you get, so if you focus on what you don't want, that's what you'll get! Any doubts or anxieties about your goal are reminders from your unconscious mind to focus on what you want. State your goal in positive terms and keep it in your mind that way.

7 Take action. Alright, it's out in the open now. The only way to get what you want is to take action, which usually means doing something different from what you've been doing so far! Asking alone won't get you to your goal—there is no such thing as a free lunch! Decide on the steps you will take, and act on the first step immediately. You don't need to know in advance every detail about how to get there. Every journey starts with the first step and moving ahead will open up new vistas and show you new opportunities for action along the way When you take action, do so from a state of excellence. Trust in yourself and your abilities and imagine yourself to be the person who has already achieved the goal. Feels pretty good, doesn't it?

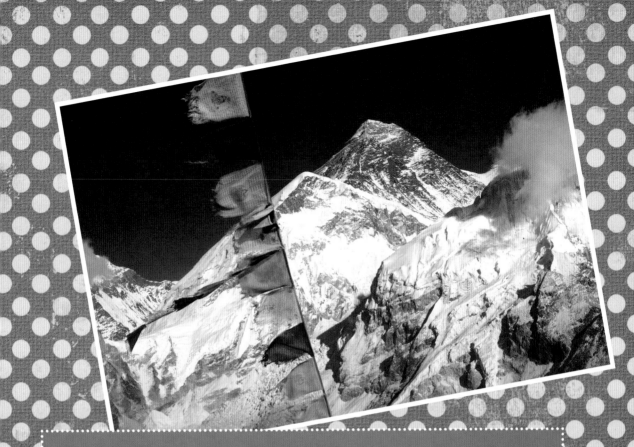

Peter Hillary (son of Sir Edmund Hillary) asserts that people, preparation and commitment are vital to achieve your own personal brand of success. And in the face of adversity, it's important to trust your own intuition. 'Up on K2 in 1995, I knew that things didn't feel right,' says Hillary, who turned away from the summit when only 400m short of it, just in time to escape a horrifying storm that took the lives of all seven of his colleagues.

Now an avid motivational speaker, Hillary encapsulates his life quest for adventure through his 'Climb Your Own Everest' teachings, listing 10 basics steps to the Summit of the World:

1. Nothing ventured, nothing gained
2. Challenge = uncertainty = excitement
3. Fear makes you focus
4. Passion gives you confidence
5. Fun makes for a great team
6. Make sure you have more than one thing to live for
7. Resist the 'flock factor'
8. You are all you have
9. Great challenges result in powerful experiences
10. A view from the summit—to new horizons

'It doesn't matter whether it is surviving a storm on a mountain, or getting your team safely through a crisis; if you survive, you live to play another day, and you will be all the stronger for the experience,' says Hillary.

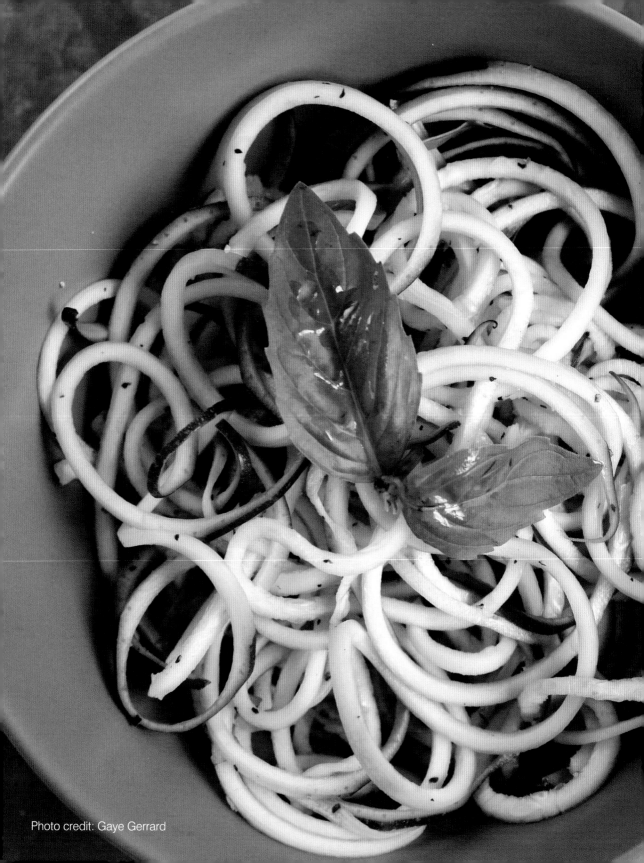

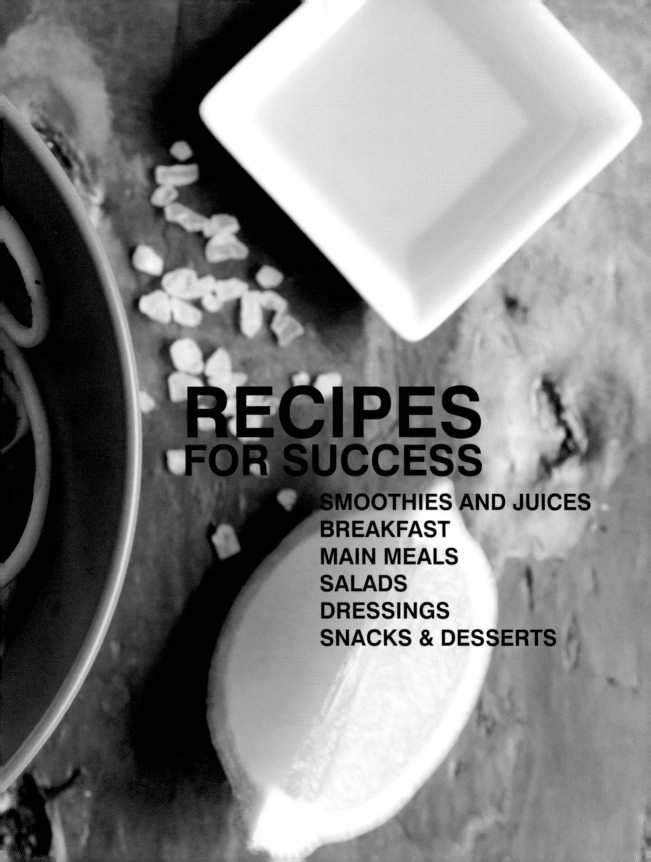

RECIPES
FOR SUCCESS

SMOOTHIES AND JUICES
BREAKFAST
MAIN MEALS
SALADS
DRESSINGS
SNACKS & DESSERTS

SMOOTHIES AND JUICES

Juices and smoothies will become your friend and 'go to' item when you need an energised boost. Whether a juice or smoothie is up to you, I love both and have either depending on the mood. Juicing takes a bit more time, where as with a smoothie I just throw the ingredients in the blender and blend. The girls from Simple Green Smoothies (simplegreensmoothies.com) have a formula I find hard to beat. Throw in some chia seeds if you want added protein or a scoop of Good Green Stuff or Clean Lean Protein if you're having as a meal. The proportions make two generous serves.

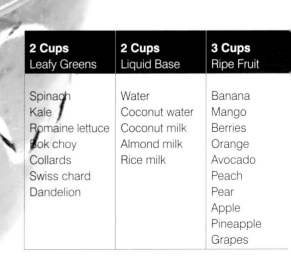

2 Cups Leafy Greens	2 Cups Liquid Base	3 Cups Ripe Fruit
Spinach	Water	Banana
Kale	Coconut water	Mango
Romaine lettuce	Coconut milk	Berries
Bok choy	Almond milk	Orange
Collards	Rice milk	Avocado
Swiss chard		Peach
Dandelion		Pear
		Apple
		Pineapple
		Grapes

KAMALAYA DETOX JUICE
Makes approximately 12 fl oz/350 mL (1 serve)

Coconut water replenishes and cools the body, while basil and pineapple support digestion—a good accompaniment to any meal. Coconut water contains electrolytes, making it a natural hydration beverage for hot climates and post-exercise training. It also aids in reducing fevers, calming the nervous system and emotional imbalances, and flushing the liver. It is a potent detoxifying agent, which neutralises toxins in the blood.

10½ fl oz/300 mL coconut water
1¾ fl oz/50 mL fresh pineapple juice
⅙ oz/5 g basil leaf

Place all ingredients in a blender with a few ice cubes and blend on medium speed until well mixed (around 30 seconds).

HIBISCUS LEMONADE
Serves 1

Rich in vitamin C and with astringent properties, this tonifying elixir also benefits the central nervous system.

2½ fl oz/80 mL hibiscus infusion *
9 fl oz/250 mL fresh pineapple juice
⅔ fl oz/20 mL lime juice

Blend the hibiscus infusion, pineapple juice and lime juice with a few ice cubes for about 30 seconds on a medium speed. Serve in a tall glass.

*To make hisbiscus infusion, take a handful of dried hibiscus flowers and simmer for 5 to 10 minutes in 10½ fl oz/300 mL of water.

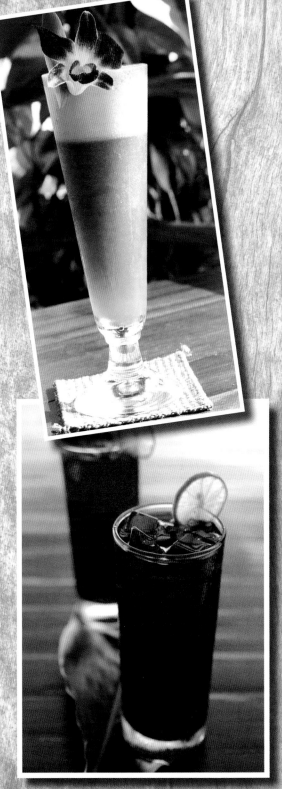

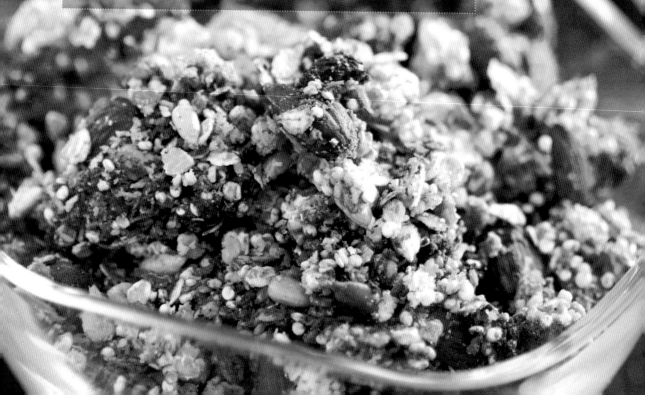

BREAKFAST

HEALTHY HOME-MADE MAPLE NUT GRANOLA

2 cups raw, whole rolled oats
1 cup sliced raw almonds
½ cup shredded coconut
¼ cup raw sunflower seeds
¼ cup raw sesame seeds
2 tbsp maple syrup (100% maple syrup, preferably grade b)
1 tbsp cinnamon
1 tsp coconut oil (a.k.a. coconut butter)
¼ tsp vanilla extract
1 large pinch fine sea salt

Combine all ingredients in a mixing bowl and mix well with your hands so everything is coated. Don't worry if the coconut oil is solid, the heat from your hands will melt it down. Spread the mixture onto a baking sheet and bake in a moderate oven for 10 minutes, until very lightly toasted. Let it cool and it can be stored in a jar in the fridge (or somewhere cool) for up to two weeks.

Eat plain, with some berries, a dollop of Greek yohgurt or a splash of almond milk—whatever makes your taste buds sing.

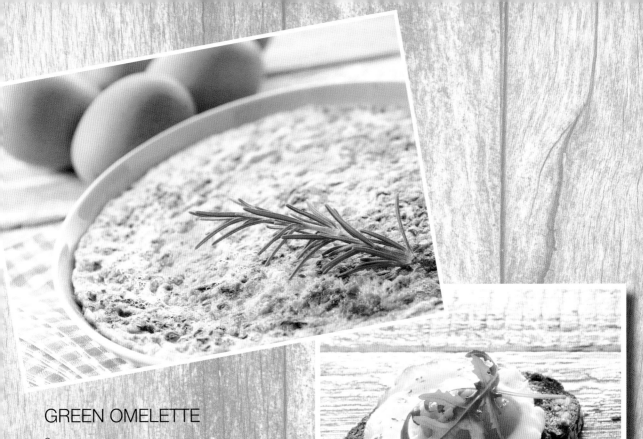

GREEN OMELETTE

2 eggs
1 cup green herbs and vegetables (spinach,
parsley, chives, basil etc.)
1 tbsp cold-pressed olive oil
1 small pinch fine sea salt
pepper to taste

Beat eggs in a bowl and finely chop greens. Use
a small amount of olive oil in a pan. Pour in egg
mixture and once bottom of omlette is set, sprinkle
greens over the top. Fold the omlette so the heat
slightly cooks the greens. Serve with blanched
spinach, mushrooms, tomoato and salt and
pepper to taste.

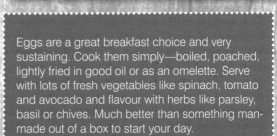

Eggs are a great breakfast choice and very
sustaining. Cook them simply—boiled, poached,
lightly fried in good oil or as an omelette. Serve
with lots of fresh vegetables like spinach, tomato
and avocado and flavour with herbs like parsley,
basil or chives. Much better than something man-
made out of a box to start your day.

MAIN MEALS

EGGPLANT MOUSSAKA ON SPINACH WITH ROASTED TOMATO SAUCE

1 large (14 oz/400 g) eggplant/aubergine, sliced 1 cm thick
1½ large (21 oz/600 g) sweet potato, 1 cm thick
2 medium (5 oz/150 g) zucchini/courgette, sliced
½ cup (3½ oz/100 g) quinoa (raw weight)
½ cup (3½ oz/100 g) green lentils (raw weight)
1 bunch English spinach, washed
sea salt and pepper

Roasted Tomato Sauce
1 lb/500 g ripe tomatoes, chopped
1 medium onion, chopped
1–2 cloves garlic, crushed
sea salt, pepper, oregano, basil
1–2 bay leaves, sprig rosemary
½ cup (3½ fl oz/100 mL) filtered water

Sprinkle eggplant with sea salt, and leave for 20–30 minutes. Rinse and dry. Pre-bake all sliced vegetables on a tray.
  Cook rinsed quinoa at a ratio of 1 cup seeds to 2 cups water on low heat and covered until all water is absorbed. Soak lentils for 2–3 hours, rinse and boil in fresh water.
  Mix quinoa and lentils with some of the tomato sauce. Stack in layers in baking dish, starting with sweet potato and finishing with a layer of eggplant.
  Bake at 160ºC for approximately 30–40 minutes, covering half way through cooking time.
If necessary, rest before cutting into squares.
  Serve on spinach leaves with extra tomato sauce and top with a dollop of cashew cheese or pesto.
  For the tomato sauce: roast tomatoes, onions and garlic in oven until they get some colour. Add spices, herbs and water. Simmer for 15–20 minutes and blend in food processor.
  Adjust seasoning to taste.

Serves 5

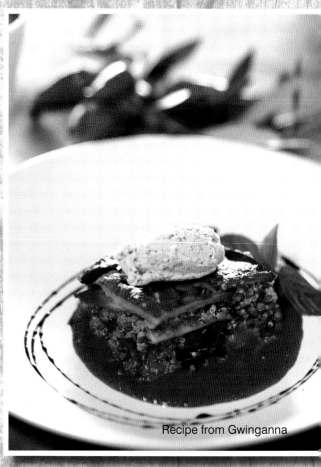

Recipe from Gwinganna

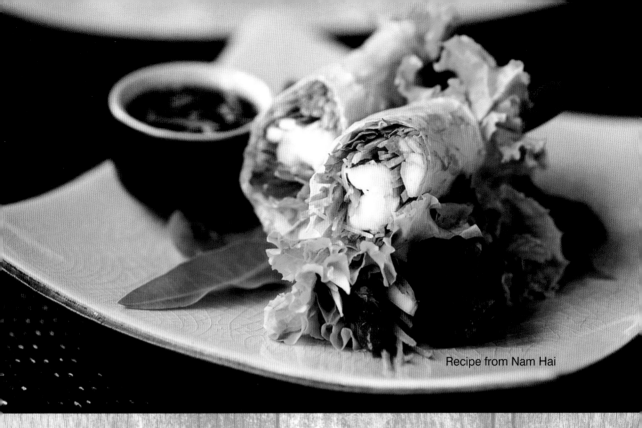

Recipe from Nam Hai

VEGETABLE AND SHRIMP/ PRAWN SPRING ROLLS

16 medium-sized poached shrimp/prawns
16 dried rice paper sheets (nam bo)
16 big lettuce leaves
1 medium size cucumber cut in thin strips
1 medium size carrot cut in thin strips
1 big handful dried rice vermicelli noodles
(soaked in hot water)
fresh herbs sprigs (mint, basil and cilantro/
coriander)
4 scallions/spring onions, chopped
1 tsp sesame seeds
salt and pepper to taste
sweet and sour fish sauce

Peel, wash and devein the poached prawns.
 Take a rice paper sheet and make it damp with
a little warm water, so it gets flexible. Repeat the
same handling with a second rice paper sheet and
place it half over the first rice paper sheet.
 Soak the dried vermicelli noodles in hot tap
water for 10–15 minutes, until softened. Drain
the noodles in a colander. Place the lettuce onto
the rice paper sheets and arrange the carrot,
cucumber, vermicelli noodles, herbs and poached
prawns evenly on top. Sprinkle some sesame
seeds on top and roll tightly to make a spring roll.
 Cut the spring roll in half and serve with sweet
and sour fish sauce on the side (recipe at
krisabbey.com).

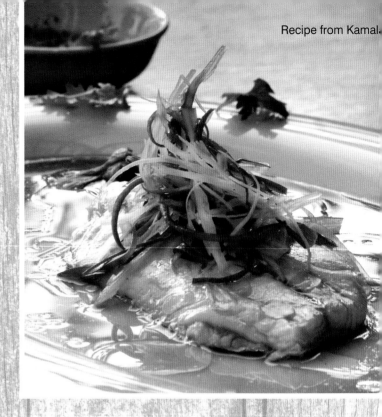

POACHED SEA BASS WITH SOY & THAI SEAFOOD SAUCE

2 fillets sea bass fillet
1 oz/30 g ginger
1 oz/30 g celery
1 oz/30 g scallions/spring onion
½ oz/15 g red chilli
6 oz/180 g soya sauce mix (below)
pinch sea salt and black pepper
9 fl oz/250 mL vegetable stock
3½ fl oz/100 mL Thai seafood sauce
 (below)
1½ fl oz/40 ml sesame oil
²/₃ fl oz/20 ml lime juice
1 bay leaf

Soya Sauce Mix
3½ oz/100 g carrot, with skin
3½ oz/100 g celery
3½ oz/100 g brown onion
3½ fl oz/100 mL soy sauce
1½ fl oz/40 mL white soya sauce
10½ fl oz/300 mL vegetable stock

Thai Seafood Sauce
5 fl oz/150 mL fish sauce, organic
5 fl oz/150 mL lime juice
4 garlic clove, finely chopped
3 chilli, finely chopped
1 tbsp palm sugar
2 tsp cilantro/coriander root, finely chopped

Begin by preparing the Soya Sauce Mix, an hour before you need it. Cut all vegetables into 2 in/5 cm slices. Place all ingredients into a wide pot and simmer on a low temperature for 1 hour. Strain the liquid, discard vegetables. Store the liquid in the refrigerator until you need it. (You can also freeze any left over and use later.)

Prepare the Thai Seafood Sauce by placing all ingredients in a blender for 1–2 minutes. Place mixture into serving bowl.

Now you're ready to prepare the fish. Cut the ginger, celery and scallions in fine strips. Heat the vegetable stock in a saucepan to a very light simmer and season with the bay leaf, celery, lime juice and sea salt. Place the fish into pan and poach for 7–10 minutes.

Meanwhile, heat the soya sauce mix and the sesame oil in separate small saucepans.

Once the fish is cooked, remove from saucepan. (Don't discard the stock. You can refrigerate or freeze it and use for soup.)

To serve, place the cooked fish fillet with skin side up on the plate and put the vegetables strips on top. Drizzle with the warmed soya sauce, followed by a drizzle of the hot sesame oil. Serve with Thai Seafood Sauce on the side.

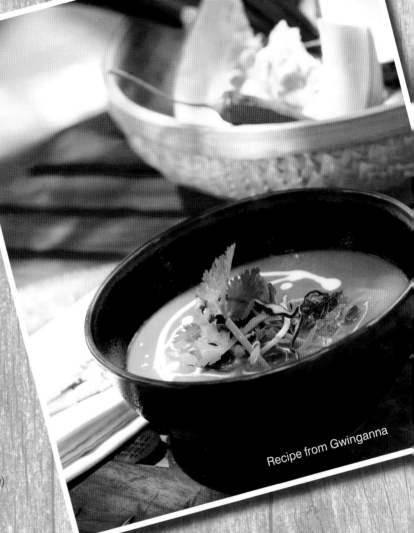

Recipe from Gwinganna

ASIAN STYLE THAI PUMPKIN SOUP

1 lb/500 g pumpkin, chopped
1 medium sweet potato, chopped
1 large onion, diced
88 fl oz/2.5 litres vegetable stock (below)
2 cloves garlic, chopped
1 knob ginger, chopped
sea salt and pepper
pinch nutmeg
1 tbsp curry powder
½ cup each carrot, zucchini/courgette, parsnip and celery, shredded
½ cup bean sprouts
4 kaffir lime leaves
¼ bunch cilantro/coriander chopped

Sauté pumpkin, sweet potato, onion and garlic with a little vegetable stock. Add spices, rest of stock and simmer for 30–40 minutes. Purée soup in a blender and check seasoning. Add the shredded vegetables just before serving and sprinkle with chopped cilantro/coriander.
 To make vegetable stock: combine trimmings including pumpkin skins, sweetcorn cobs, carrots, onions and celery (no leaves, they make the stock bitter) with 3 litres of filtered water. Add a bay leaf or two, some peppercorns and a pinch of sea salt and boil for about 30 minutes. Strain.

Serves 8

SALADS

SOM TAM

Thailand's green papaya salad combines the four main tastes of Thai cuisine: sour lime, hot chilli, salty fish sauce, and sweetness added by palm sugar. As the green papaya is not ripe, it has a slightly tart flavour that works well with the spice of chilli and the saltiness of fish sauce, as well as the sweetness of honey. The good news continues as this salad is easy to make, is low in calories and high in fibre. It can be served alone or with other Thai-style dishes.

3 cups green papaya, cut into long thin juliennes
1 or 2 long beans, cut into 3 cm pieces
2 cloves garlic
5–10 small green or red bird's eye chillies
2 tbsp lime juice
1 tbsp light soy sauce or fish sauce
1 tsp palm sugar or honey
3 tomatoes, sliced into segments
1 tbsp jungle peanuts or cashews, roasted or raw
½ cup carrots, shredded (optional)

Pound the garlic and chilies in a large mortar; add the long beans and pound again lightly.

Add the other ingredients and mix all by lightly mashing in the mortar. Do not make the ingredients mushy.

When serving, top with cashews or almonds. If the salad is served as a course by itself, it may be accompanied with a selection of sliced vegetables such as cabbage, long beans, cucumbers and lettuce. Garnish with ¼ cup chopped cashew nuts.

Serves 4–6

Experiment with salads. Pile your plate high with a rainbow of fresh ingredients and a good dressing. Even lettuce and tomato can be jazzed up with a sprinkle of crushed walnuts, a drizzle of good oil and a squeeze of lemon juice. Now that's my idea of fast food!

CORIANDER IS A GREAT GARNISH OR ADDITION TO MANY SOUPS AND SALADS. IT AIDS DIGESTION AS IT SPEEDS UP FOOD MOVEMENT FROM THE STOMACH. IT'S KNOWN TO HAVE HEAVY METAL CHELATING PROPERTIES TOO!

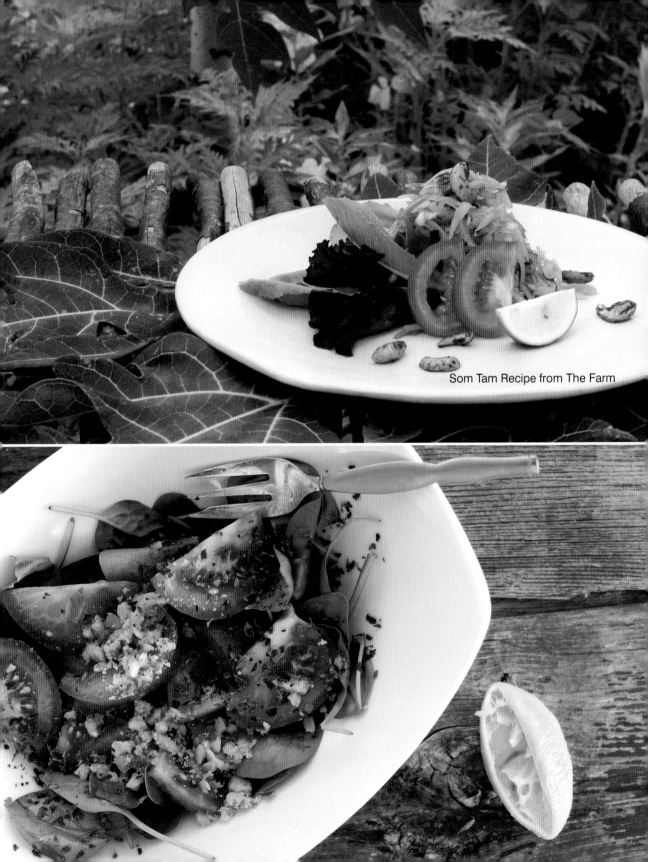

Som Tam Recipe from The Farm

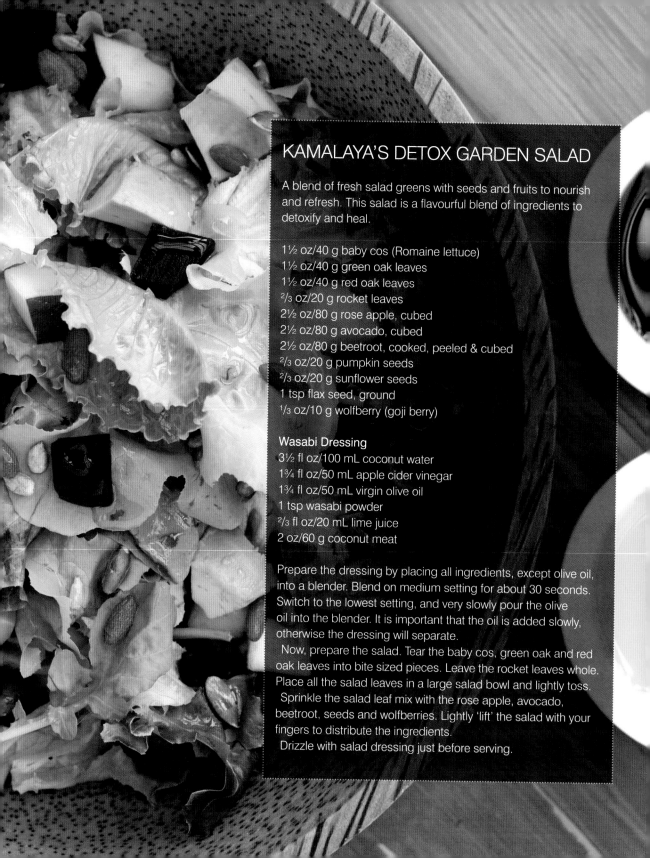

KAMALAYA'S DETOX GARDEN SALAD

A blend of fresh salad greens with seeds and fruits to nourish and refresh. This salad is a flavourful blend of ingredients to detoxify and heal.

1½ oz/40 g baby cos (Romaine lettuce)
1½ oz/40 g green oak leaves
1½ oz/40 g red oak leaves
⅔ oz/20 g rocket leaves
2½ oz/80 g rose apple, cubed
2½ oz/80 g avocado, cubed
2½ oz/80 g beetroot, cooked, peeled & cubed
⅔ oz/20 g pumpkin seeds
⅔ oz/20 g sunflower seeds
1 tsp flax seed, ground
⅓ oz/10 g wolfberry (goji berry)

Wasabi Dressing
3½ fl oz/100 mL coconut water
1¾ fl oz/50 mL apple cider vinegar
1¾ fl oz/50 mL virgin olive oil
1 tsp wasabi powder
⅔ fl oz/20 mL lime juice
2 oz/60 g coconut meat

Prepare the dressing by placing all ingredients, except olive oil, into a blender. Blend on medium setting for about 30 seconds. Switch to the lowest setting, and very slowly pour the olive oil into the blender. It is important that the oil is added slowly, otherwise the dressing will separate.

Now, prepare the salad. Tear the baby cos, green oak and red oak leaves into bite sized pieces. Leave the rocket leaves whole. Place all the salad leaves in a large salad bowl and lightly toss.

Sprinkle the salad leaf mix with the rose apple, avocado, beetroot, seeds and wolfberries. Lightly 'lift' the salad with your fingers to distribute the ingredients.

Drizzle with salad dressing just before serving.

DRESSINGS

Having a good salad dressing on hand takes any salad from 'so so' to sensational. Teresa Cutter has a bunch of great recipes on her site thehealthychef.com, here is one of them:

BALSAMIC HONEY AND WALNUT DRESSING

¼ cup aged balsamic vinegar
2 tsp Dijon mustard
2 tsp honey
2 tbsp finely chopped roasted walnuts
2 tbsp cold pressed olive oil or walnut oil (optional)

Combine all the ingredients.
Add the oil if you need a milder flavoured dressing.
Store in the fridge for up to five days.
Delicious with baby spinach leaves and nuts.

BEST ZESTY DRESSING

This is one of my recipes that has some kick.

¼ cup red wine vinegar
juice from 1 lime
juice from 1 lemon
1 tsp finely chopped chilli
2 tsp honey
2 tbsp finely chopped cilantro/coriander
2 tbsp cold pressed olive oil
salt and pepper to taste

Combine in a jar and give a good shake. This lasts in the fridge for a good five days. This is great with any salad of a Thai nature, and especially good with avocado.

SNACKS & DESSERTS

CHOCOLATE PECAN PIE

Crust
½ cup almonds, soaked for 8 hours and
 dehydrated until crispy
1½ cups pecan nuts, soaked and dehydrated
6 dates, pitted
¼ cup muscovado sugar
½ tsp cinnamon

Chocolate
¾ cup cocoa powder
¾ cup honey
⅓ cup coconut oil, warmed

Filling
½ cup coconut butter
¾ cup dates, pitted
2 tbsp maple syrup
1 tbsp vanilla extract
1¼ cups pecan nuts, chopped

Topping
1 cup candied pecans (see recipe below)

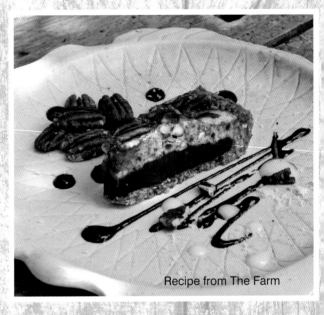

Recipe from The Farm

CANDIED PECANS
2 kg pecan nuts, soaked
1½ cups maple syrup
5 tbsp cinnamon powder
1 tsp salt
pinch nutmeg

In a bowl, combine all ingredients and mix
thoroughly.
 Cover with a cloth and marinate overnight.
 Pour into a dehydrator tray with a teflex sheet
and dehydrate at 90°C for 24 hours.
 Transfer to a sterilised clear jar and store in
freezer. Can last for 1 to 2 months.

For crust, place almonds, pecans, dates, sugar
and cinnamon in a food processor; process until
crumbly, yet, sticky. Press mixture firmly into a
9-inch pie plate lined with cling film or greaseproof
paper and set aside.
 Mix the chocolate ingredients together, then blend
in a high-speed blender to achieve a smooth
consistency. Pour ¾ of a cup of the mixture into
the pie crust and refrigerate until firm (approx.
2 hours). Save the chocolate mixture that remains
for chocolate truffles.
 For filling, place the dates and coconut oil in a
food processor and blend until smooth. Add the
rest of the ingredients and continue to blend until
smooth. Fold in the chopped pecans by hand and
spread on top of the chilled chocolate bottom.
 Arrange nuts in symmetrical fashion around the
edge of the pie and chill the pie for minimum of
four hours before serving.

PINEAPPLE LEMONGRASS SKEWERS

5 oz/150 g fresh pineapple
1 g lemongrass fresh
1 g fresh chilli
2 g fresh mint
9 g lemongrass stick
2 ml lime juice
Mint Essence
1¾ fl oz/50 ml pineapple juice
2 oz/60 g young coconut mix
a few mint leaves
a few drops of lime juice

Cut the pineapple in 3 equal sized pieces.
 Chop the chilli and lemongrass very fine. Rub the pineapple with the chopped lemongrass and chilli (be easy on the chilli).
 Skew the pineapple on the skewers and heat up the pan, roast quickly each side in the pan until golden brown, then place on a paper towel.
 Cut the mint in julienne and sprinkle on top of the skewers. Serve with mint essence.
 For the mint essence, place all ingredients in to a blender and mix well on a medium level. Serve.

RAW DATE AND ALMOND SLICE

1 cup almonds, soaked overnight, discard water
2 cups dates, soaked for a couple of hours (1 cup for topping)
1 cup filtered water
½ cup carob powder
2 cups coconut meat or dessicated coconut

Add the soaked almonds, 1 cup of dates, filtered water and carob. Blend in a food processor until smooth.
 Mix in the coconut, then press the mix into a biscuit tray, to about 1 inch thickness. Leave covered in the fridge for 2–3 hours to firm up.
 For the topping: process the second cup of dates in blender with a little water until smooth like a 'cake icing' and spread over the set mix. Sprinkle with some coconut or other nuts of your choice.
 Rest in the fridge, then cut into small squares to serve.

Makes 20 squares

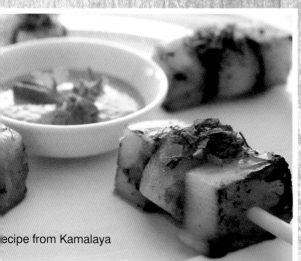
ecipe from Kamalaya

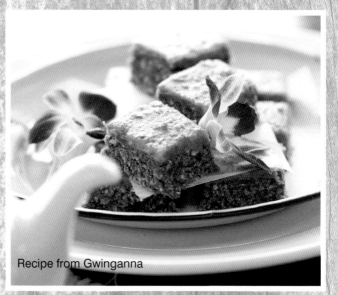
Recipe from Gwinganna

DETOX SPAS

In my role as editor of *Spa Life* magazine, I am fortunate enough to visit some of the most incredible destination spas around the world in the name of work! Four of the best were kind enough to allow me to share some of their special detox recipes with you. If this book inspires you to take the next step with your health, with my hand on my heart, I would say get to one of these places. You will experience something life-changing and magical!

One of the most incredible places I have been is Vietnam, more specifically is Hoi An. I stayed at the Nam Hai, which is situated right on the beach and a short (but a scary) bike ride from the UNESCO heritage listed village of Hoi An. The spa, food and people make you want to go back again and again.
thenamhai.com

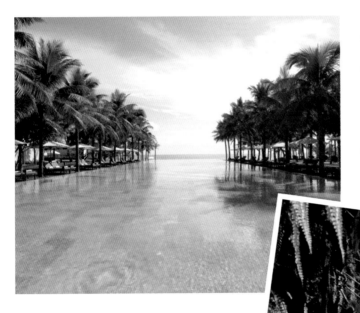

The Farm at San Benito in the Philippines was one of the very first destination retreats I experienced. It is a must do. The food was an absolute highlight. It was my first real experience of eating raw food. Who would have thought chocolate cake could be that good (and raw). The grounds are a secluded paradise. Very fond memories of this place.
thefarmatsanbenito.com

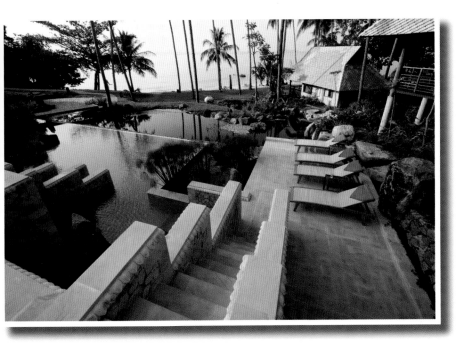

Kamalaya is a multi-award winning wellness sanctuary and holistic spa on the tropical southern coastline of Koh Samui, offering inspired healthy cuisine alongside a choice of tailored wellness programmes including detox, stress and burnout and personalised yoga. It is the brainchild of John and Karina Stewart, who ooze nourish and nurture from every pore of their bodies.
kamalaya.com.

Gwinganna is just one of those places that every person in Australia should visit, in fact your health fund should susidise your stay. It is truly life-changing. You will not only get back to nature, but you will get back to you! The food is so nourishing, tasty and literally paddock to plate. It is up there as one of the best in the world!
gwinganna.com

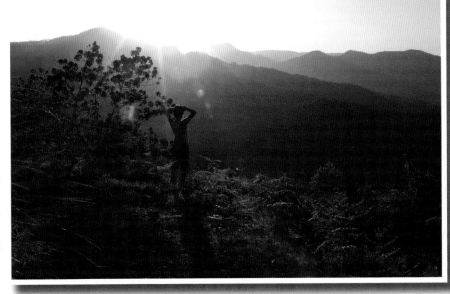

RESOURCES

BOOKS I RECOMMEND

Ancient Wisdom For Modern Health by Mark Bunn (Enlightened Health Publishing)

Anything by Patrick Holford Mark Sisson or James Duigan (Those guys are geniuses)

Authentic Woman: A Guide to Beauty, Body & Bliss by Leslie & Susannah Kenton (Vermillon)

Clean & Lean Diet: 14 Days to Your Best Ever Body by James Duigan (Kyle Cathie Limited)

Detox: Regaining Your Health & Vitality by Penelope Sach (Penguin)

Detox: Your Guide to Detox by Metagenics (Health World Limited)

Food Glorious Food: Incredibly delicious Low GI Recipes by Patrick Holford & Fiona McDonald (Piatkus)

Recipes for Health BlissL Using Nature Foods & Lifestyle Choices to Rejuvenate Your Body & Life by Susan Smith Jones, PhD (Hay House)

The Primal Blue Print by Mark Sisson (Vermilion)

The Reboot with Joe Juice Diet by Joe Cross (Hodder & Stoughton)

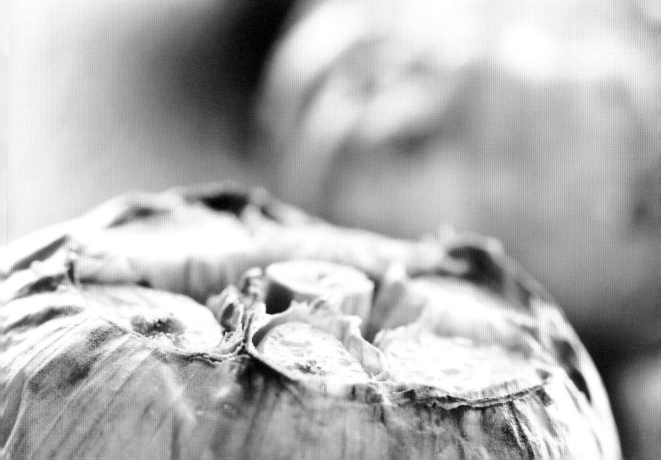

WEBSITES I LOVE

thehealthychef.com (Awesome healthy recipes using Low HI & real food)

foodhealthwealth.com (Sam Gowing makes some of the best raw food I've tasted)

simplegreensmoothies.com (The best smoothie recipes you'll find)

sweetlyraw.com (For all the sweet teeth out there ... this site satisfies)

krisabbey.com (Have to)

goop.com (Just do)

themiddlefingerproject.org (For good advice shot from the hip)

spaandbewell.com (of course!)

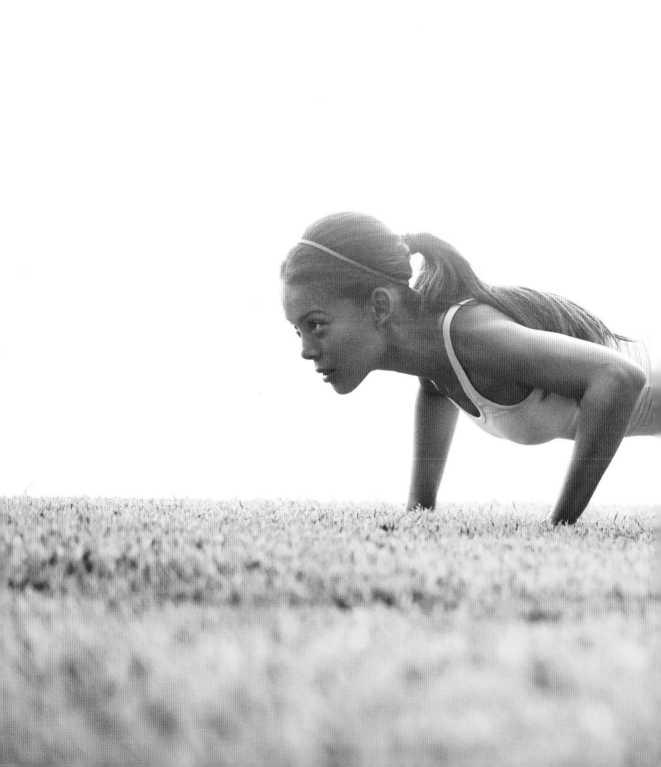

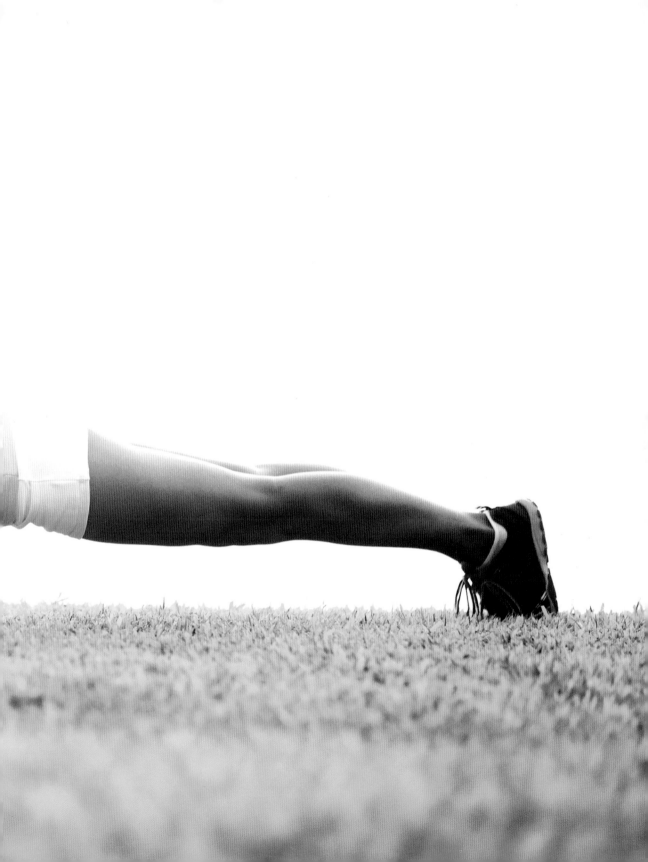

I first embarked on Kris's "Get Clean Get Lean" program May 2011. I can honestly say, that with the support she gave, together with the food suggestions and exercise advice, it turned my life around. I lost 4kg which have stayed off and I have become much more mindful of my food choices. I now make the decision to get back in line with the detox program each year, as it feels so good to do so. I have consistently lost 2kg each time. I have always loved cooking and now just have a wider choice of wonderful foods, my entire relationship with sweet and sugary foods has changed for the better. I would encourage anyone to give it a go. All you have to lose is a bit of weight and a heap of wonderful feelings to gain. ~ Julie Coulson

This detox by far was the most simple and enjoyable detox I have ever done, throughout the 4 weeks I enjoyed cooking so many different foods which made me feel alive! I lost 5kg and learnt so much from it. Such as; how much sugar (especially processed) badly effects your mind, sleep and energy levels when you eat it and how much better everything feels when you don't! I had great support from Kris and loved every minute of it! My biggest problem before the detox was the amount of bread that I ate...now I barely touch it because I have found other ways to compensate and keep me full for longer to stop me just eating bread as an easy-fix meal! I will continue eating like this for the rest of my life! ~ Jenna Patterson